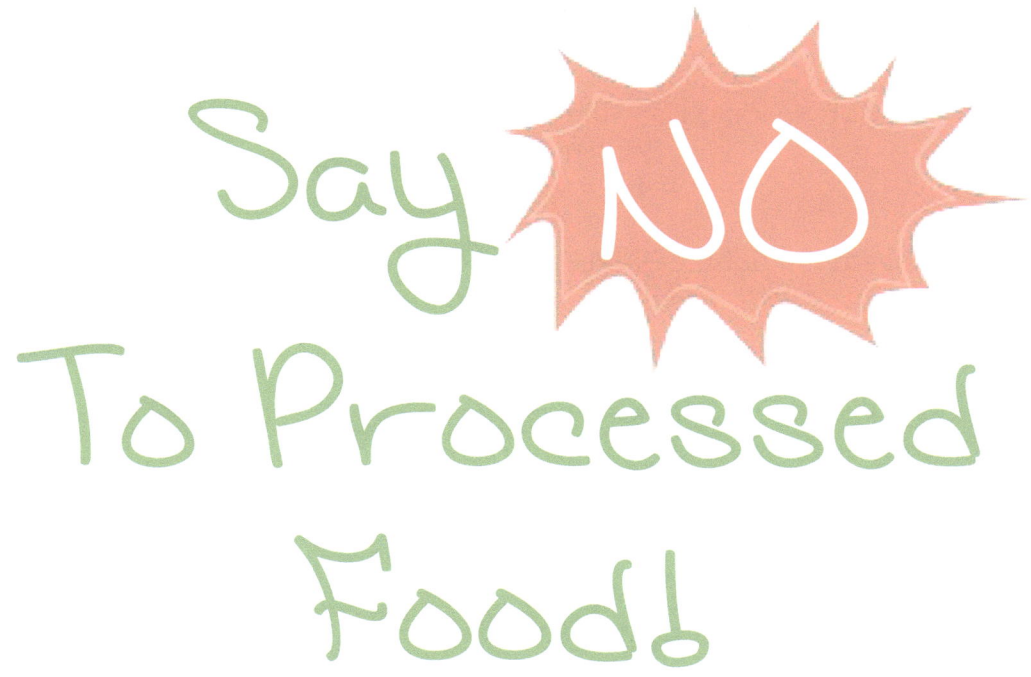

Say NO To Processed Food!

A clean eating recipe book that will give you a healthier life

- No More Preservatives
- No More Artificial Flavoring
- Clean Eating

J. J. Lewis

Want more Bestseller Cook Books for **FREE?**

Join my **V.I.P** Reading List where I give away **Healthy** and Delicious Recipes **FOR FREE!**

Yes, you heard me right! COMPLETELY FREE to everyone just for being a loyal reader of mine!

www.ravenspress.com/jjlewis

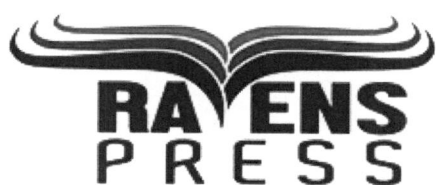

RAVENS PRESS

ISBN-13: 978-1516935901

ISBN-10: 151693590X

www.amazon.com/author/jjlewis

TABLE OF CONTENTS

INTRODUCTION

If you are a health enthusiast, you have probably heard of clean eating as a new form of diet. Clean eating does not literally mean eating foods that are not dirty. Clean eating could mean a number of things—from eating foods that have no artificial ingredients to eating foods that have not been processed or refined. Many experts believe that clean eating is the best way to improve your health because you are eating natural foods that do not contain any harmful chemicals and have not undergone processes that can cause changes in the food's nutritional composition.

For those living really unhealthy and inactive lifestyles, hearing about the concept of clean eating is like being given a death sentence. They treat this as a scare tactic to get them to move their bodies, start exercising and decreasing their total daily food intake. But in reality, clean eating should be that right kind of motivation for them to embark on a quest of finding and rediscovering their best selves.

The Clean Eating Cookbook is the perfect ally that you should have to make sure that you will be able to properly take on the challenge of giving your pantry, grocery list, your cooking and your food choices complete makeovers. How? Well, the book offers you tons of helpful bits of information, which can be very beneficial in ensuring that you will not only lose the weight that you have been trying to shed for many years, at the same time, you and your family will feel more energetic and will soon achieve the best state of health.

Chapter 1: What is Clean Eating?

Contrary to what most people believe, this practice is not a diet. But rather, clean eating is a lifestyle. This is not something that you can follow just to lose weight and forego once you have achieved your weight loss goals. Eating clean is a practice that you and your family should ultimately live by for the rest of your lives.

The concept of clean eating has been practiced ever since the first man learned how to make use of the natural vegetation and wild animal resources in their areas. It is simply eating organic, lean and naturally obtained fruits, vegetables and meat using the simplest and the healthiest preparations.
To better understand what this healthy lifestyle is all about, you definitely need to find out more about its principles.

This is because you need to make some major changes in your life, especially if you have been leading an unhealthy lifestyle by eating mostly junk foods, processed foods, or instant meals. Clean eating is not the same as those diet fads that promise to help you lose weight. This is more about improving the quality of food that you eat than limiting the quantity. It also has something to do with changing your eating habits and your lifestyle.

Most of the food items included in the clean eating diet plan are also recommended by public health groups and organizations. Compared to diet fads, clean eating is more flexible and can be adapted to almost all kinds of lifestyle.

To help you understand what clean eating is, you need to know the basic principles of clean eating. Check out the paragraphs below.

Principles of clean eating

Whole Foods is the Best

Whole foods are foods that have not been processed and are in their most natural state. For example, whole grains are grains that still contain all the original layers or parts including the endosperm, germ, and bran. Grains that are crushed, cracked, or rolled are already considered processed. Natural foods are those that do not have any chemicals or artificial ingredients in them. Whole natural foods contain all the nutrients that are found in the original nutritional value of the food.

Unrefined vs. Refined Foods

Refined foods are processed foods that no longer have all the nutrients that they originally had. Certain foods have to undergo this process to improve their taste, give them a longer shelf life, and create a finer appearance and texture. One example is refined white sugar. It is best to choose unrefined brown sugar than white sugar for in your coffee or tea. However, when it comes to baking, most recipes require the use of white sugar because it gives a smoother and silkier texture to the bread or pastry. But if you want to get the complete nutrients of the food, you have to make sure that you choose unrefined over refined food products

Gives You the Cooking Independence

Meals prepared at home are known and proven to be several times healthier than your favorite fast food meals. No matter how much these restaurants claim that they use nothing but the best products, you can never be too sure that they do not use processed food products. Clean eating will help you learn how to prepare fast, simple and healthy meals.

Consume more Fruits and Vegetables

One thing that all diet plans and diet fads have in common is that all of them promote eating more fruits and vegetables. Everyone knows how beneficial fruits and vegetables are to your health. They contain vitamins and minerals that your body needs without having to worry about adding more calories. Fruits and vegetables also make you feel full longer, which prevents you from overeating. When choosing fruits and vegetables, be sure to pick those that came directly from the farm. You can buy fresh fruits and vegetables from your local farmer's market or stalls that sell produce.

Consume less saturated fats.

Fats in general are not bad ftor your health, contrary to popular belief. However, there is a specific kind of fats that you need to avoid called saturated fats. These fats are found in dairy products and meat. Clean eating does not mean that you should completely eliminate fats from your diet; in fact, that is not recommended because fats are also important to your health. What you need is to focus on good fats such as those found in canola oil, olive oil, nuts, and fish.

Lesser sodium Intake.

The daily recommendation for sodium is only 2300 mg per day and most Americans eat 1,000 mg more sodium than the limit because they often eat fast foods and processed foods. To ensure that your sodium intake is still within the limit, you should consider eating out less frequently and cooking your own food at home. You can make your meals tastier even without adding too much salt by using spices and herbs.

Reduce Meat Consumption.

Meat has saturated fats that are bad for your health. However, you cannot completely eliminate meat from your diet because it is an important source of protein. What you can do is to use meat as flavoring to your meals instead of serving it as the meal itself. For example, instead of eating fried chicken for dinner, you should consider adding bits of chicken in your soup.

No to high calorie drinks.

Instead of drinking soft drinks or specialty coffees that are high in calories, you should consider drinking plain water instead. In the morning, you can drink low-fat skim milk, unsweetened tea, or freshly squeezed fruit juice for breakfast.

Eat 5 to 6 small meals in a day.

The clean eating diet plan encourages people to eat small meals, about five to six times a day instead of eating two or three large meals. Skipping meals is not encouraged and eating healthy snacks in between meals is encouraged. This prevents you from overeating and keeps your energy level stable throughout the day.

Reduce your alcohol intake.

You can still drink alcohol but you should limit your alcohol intake and avoid getting drunk. For women, the recommended limit for alcohol is one drink per day. For men, the limit is 2 drinks per day. Too much alcohol is bad for your health because it can cause dehydration and can add calories to your diet.

No to Processed Foods

Canned, packed and labeled foods are considered to be processed types of food. The thing about such types of foods is that they may contain ingredients, such as preservatives that could be chemically laced and are harmful to your body. But if there are processed foods that you can eat, those would be whole grain pastas, vegan meat substitutes, organic grains and flours and cheeses. Every time you read the labels, keep in mind that if you cannot pronounce it, do not buy it!

Lessen your sugar intake.

Aside from sodium, you should also watch your sugar intake. The recommended sugar intake is 9 teaspoons for men and 6 teaspoons for women. You should avoid sugary foods like baked treats, candies, and soda. You should also watch out for healthy foods with added sugar like cereal, yogurt, and tomato sauce.

Right Combination of Carbs and Protein is the Key

This will encourage you to go for more balanced meals every single day. Whether you are snacking or having lunch, your plate should have the right proportions of carbs and protein. This will not only make your healthier, you will also be able to quell all your bouts of hunger and unrealistic cravings.

Chapter 2: Benefits of Clean Eating

Because of the kinds of food that you are encouraged to eat with the clean eating diet plan, you can get a lot of benefits that help improve your health. Some of the benefits of eating clean are listed in the paragraphs below.

Energy Booster

Getting the right kind and amount of nutrients helps boost your energy. For example, iron and vitamin B-complex improves cellular functions. Clean eating also promotes eating small meals more frequently. This helps regulate the sugar level in your blood stream which gives you a steady supply of energy throughout the day. This is also due to your reduced consumption of sweets and refined carbohydrates.

Improves your digestive system's processes

Have you noticed that after eating that large serving of cheese burger and a handful of fries, your stomach feels so full and totally acidic? Well, if you observe carefully, you will even hear your digestive enzymes struggle to work their way through all the oily processed foods that you have consumed. Clean eating will help put a stop to acid refluxes, indigestion and poor bowel movement. You will have all the fiber that you need to improve your digestion in so many ways.

Lose Weight Effectively

The kinds of food that you eat also help you lose weight if you practice clean eating. also help you lose weight. For instance, it promotes low sugar intake that helps you achieve optimum weight. It also encourages you to eat more fruits and vegetables and less meat which lowers your calorie intake. Aside from eating healthy foods, clean eating also promotes an active lifestyle. You can do some exercises or be more physically active that can help you lose weight.

Lessen the feeling of Hunger

Junk food makes you crave more food, which in turn makes you gain those unwanted pounds. Eating cleaner and healthier food will make sure that you will feel full and satisfied longer since you will be completely nourished.

Boost Immunity

Eating clean foods also protects you against diseases like heart diseases, stroke, diabetes, and cancer. It helps lower your cholesterol level and boosts the strength of your blood vessels. Fruits and vegetables are also rich in vitamins and minerals that promote strong immunity that helps you fight illnesses. And because you are eating less saturated fat, the cholesterol level in your body is also regulated. The artificial and chemical ingredients in processed foods also increase risk of cancer. Fruits and vegetables are rich in antioxidants and phytonutrients that are known to help fight cancer cells.

Cooking is more fun

This lifestyle does not mean that you have to eat bland and dull looking meals every single time. Clean eating, with all the amazingly healthy ingredients that you can choose from, should and will encourage you to try new recipes to bring life to your dishes. Clean eating should get you excited to prepare your own meals!

Mental Health Improver

Aside from improving your physical health, eating clean foods also helps boost your mental health. Fish is rich in omega-3 fatty acids, a good kind of fat included in the clean eating diet plan. This fat helps fight depression and moodiness. Vitamin B-6, which can be found in sunflower seeds, pistachio nuts, and tuna, also helps produce dopamine, a hormone in the body that makes you feel good and happy.

Good for Everyone

Gone are the days when you think that healthy or clean eating is just for vegans, vegetarians, diabetes, heart patients or those who are on a really strict diet. Clean eating is for those who would like to take great care of themselves better.

Skin Enhancer

If you are healthy from within, your outward appearance will also look healthy which includes your hair and skin. Some fruits and vegetables are rich in antioxidants that are known to fight wrinkles and skin blemishes. Fruits and vegetables also have higher water content, which keeps your skin hydrated at all times. You also do not have to worry about chemicals that can be harmful to your body and can cause damage to your skin.

Chapter 3: Clean Eating Tips That Will You Lose Weight Effectively

It is important that you know some useful tips that will help you lose weight and rejuvenate. You also need to know some tips on how to make clean and green eating a permanent part of your life. Remember that this is not just a diet fad that you only need to do for a limited time frame. This requires significant changes in your routine and your life in general, which is why it is important that you plan the transition carefully. Here are some tips and ideas you might find useful.

Get plenty of exercise

Changing your diet alone is not enough to achieve your optimum weight and health. You also need to get the right amount of exercise that your body needs to burn the calories you get from the food you eat and prevent them from turning into fat. You need to exercise regularly if you want to lose weight and to keep yourself healthy. You can do some cardio workout and muscle and strength training that will help you lose weight and become more fit and healthy. You can either pay for a monthly gym membership where you have a personal trainer, or do the exercises yourself at the park or at home.

Aside from regular workouts, you can also get enough exercise by being more physically active. Instead of driving your car to buy a carton of milk at the grocery just a couple of blocks away from your house, you should consider walking or riding your bike. Instead of using the elevator, you can use the stairs to go to your office floor, unless of course your office is located on the 23rd floor or something. If that's the case, you should consider riding the elevator halfway or two-thirds up, then using the stairs for the remaining few floors.

Spice Up Your Meals

Iif you are a bit scared to try new spices and seasoning blends, why don't you go for herbs and other ingredients that could elevate and take your healthy meals to whole new levels? Try experimenting and incorporating these healthy herbs and spices in your next recipes:

- Cloves
- Cinnamon
- Nutmeg
- Cumin
- Turmeric
- Sage
- Mint
- Rosemary
- Basil
- Marjoram
- Chili
- Thyme

Get enough sleep and rest

Getting enough sleep and rest is also a part of a clean lifestyle. Resting or sleeping makes your body refreshed and rejuvenated the next day. This will allow you to perform your tasks more efficiently. It is also easier to follow your clean eating lifestyle if you have enough energy. For example, you will have the energy to prepare clean meals throughout the day and do some exercises if your body is well-rested.

Plan your meals

There are several ways to diversify your meals on a daily basis. Make the internet your best friend, or this book to look for amazingly delicious, but unbelievably healthy dishes that you can easily make for your family. You can create a chart and plan what you will be cooking and eating for a week or in the next few days.

Learn the different recommendations for food groups

Clean eating is also about balanced eating. Eating whole, natural foods will be useless if you do not get the recommended amount of all the food groups. You need to know what foods are great sources of protein, carbohydrates, good fats, vitamins, minerals, fiber, and other nutrients that your body needs. It is important to get the recommended amount of each of these nutrients in your diet because they have different functions that keep you healthy and improve your general well-being. For instance, fiber's main function is to flush out toxins in your body and improve your bowel movement. Protein, on the other hand, improves your strength and muscles.

Experiment in the kitchen

Do not be afraid to get out of your comfort zone and experiment on different healthy recipes that you have found. You can try small portions first and see if you and the rest of the family will like what you have prepared.

Read the nutrition labels and ingredient list

Any health conscious individual should know how to read nutrition labels because this is where you can find the amount of nutrients that the food item contains. The nutrition label usually includes macronutrients such as protein, carbohydrates, and fats. It also includes vitamins and minerals. You will also know the calories that the food product has and the number of servings per package. It is important that you know how to read nutrition labels to ensure that you are getting the adequate amount of required nutrients.

Aside from the nutrition label, you also need to know how to read the ingredients list. One useful tip is to avoid any food item that has an ingredient whose name is too long and difficult to pronounce because it is most likely an artificial or chemical ingredient.

Cook your meals ahead

You really do not have to be a slave in the kitchen every day, because there are healthy or nutritious meals that you can make ahead of time, store in the fridge and reheat. You can even label the containers with the dates or day that they should be consumed to keep their freshness and maintain their flavors.

Get rid of vices and bad habits

Clean eating does not completely forbid you to drink alcohol but there is a recommended amount which is 1 drink for women and 2 drinks for men. You should also quit smoking and stop using illegal drugs if you want to stay healthy, lose weight, and make clean eating a permanent part of your life. Aside from these, you also need to stop doing bad habits like staying up really late at night, skipping meals, and eating fast food and takeout all the time.

Make a list

Do not get too overly excited to shop for fruits, veggies, meats and dairy products. Keep a record of what ingredients you have and take note of their expiration dates; this list will serve are your reference for the next time that you will go grocery shopping.

Stock up on clean foods

Another important tip to adoapt a clean eating habit is to stock up on clean foods like fresh fruits and vegetables, whole bread and pasta, lean meat, skinless poultry, and so on. It will be easier to follow your clean eating diet if you already have something anything to cook in your kitchen. Most of the time, people go back to their old eating habits because they do not have something to cook in their kitchen. Buying clean foods is not difficult because you can easily find them in your local grocery or market. You need to prepare a 7-day meal plan at the start of the week, so that you will know what you need to buy when you go grocery shopping. This will prevent you from going back to your old ways because you already have your meals and grocery shopping planned.

Learn how to cook

It is also easier to follow the clean eating lifestyle if you know how to cook. There may be some restaurants that offer clean foods, but they can be difficult to find. If you know how to cook, you do not have to worry about finding the right restaurant that uses clean foods for their meals. Cooking your own food also gives variety. You will get tired of eating the same foods from the local restaurant that offers clean foods in your area. You do not have to be a chef to prepare clean meals. You can use simple recipes at first before moving on to more difficult and elaborate recipes.

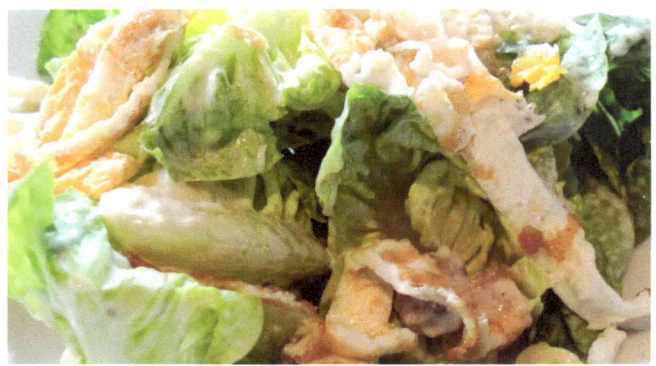

1. Fresh Salmon Salad and Crispy Potatoes

This is a healthy dish that even your kids will love. The light and fresh salmon salad has all the flavors and textures that you love—the crispiness of the potatoes, the freshness of green beans, and the tangy dressing that completes the dish. This is the perfect dish for the busy individual because it only takes about 25 minutes to prepare.

Ingredients:

• About 14 oz. salmon, bones and skin removed
• 4 cups of arugula
• 2 small potatoes, preferable yellow-fleshed like Yukon Gold (no need to peel potatoes, just scrub and slice them thinly)
• 1 medium-sized shallot, sliced thinly
• A quarter cup of buttermilk
• 2 tbsp. of extra virgin olive oil, to be used separately
• 2 tsp. of rice vinegar
• Half a tsp. of salt, to be used separately

Instructions:

1. Turn on the stove to medium-high heat and place a nonstick skillet over the burner. Heat a tbsp. of olive oil and cook potatoes until crispy and golden brown in color. This will take about 5 to 6 minutes on each side. Once cooked, put the potatoes on a plate and sprinkle with a quarter tsp of salt. It is best to serve them warm, so be sure to cover them with aluminum foil to retain the heat.

2. In a small pan, mix together the rest of the salt and olive oil with the rice vinegar and boil the mixture. Turn off the stove and remove the pan from the burner to stop the cooking process. Add the buttermilk and stir using a whisk.

3. Dress the salmon with the warm buttermilk mixture. Get 4 plates and layer your arugula leaves on each plate. Put the dressed salmon and crispy potatoes on the bed of arugula. Serve.

4. Makes 4 servings.

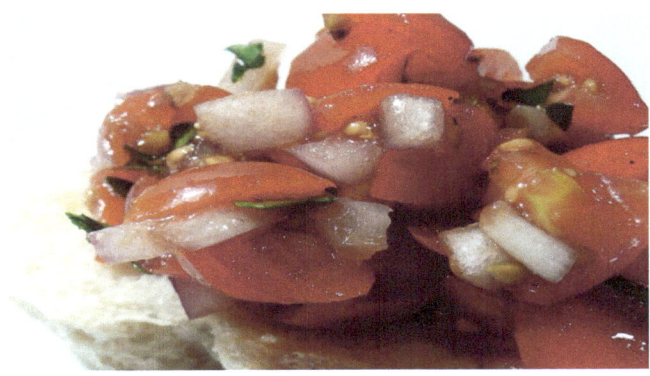

2. Balsamic Tomato Bruschetta

Ingredients:

•8 plum or Roma tomatoes de-seeded and diced
• 1/3 cup of basil chopped
• ¼ of parmesan cheese shredded
• 2 large garlic cloves minced
• 1 Tablespoons of high quality balsamic vinegar
• 1 teaspoon of olive oil
• ¼ teaspoon of sea or kosher salt
• ¼ teaspoon of black pepper
• 1 loaf of French bread sliced and toasted.

Instructions:

In a large bowl, combine tomatoes, cheese, basil and garlic together. Add in the balsamic vinegar, olive oil, salt and pepper. Cover and let the mixture marinate in the fridge for at least 30 minutes to let the flavors marry together.

Once ready to serve, toast the slices of French bread drizzled in with olive oil. Spoon the marinated tomato mixture and serve.

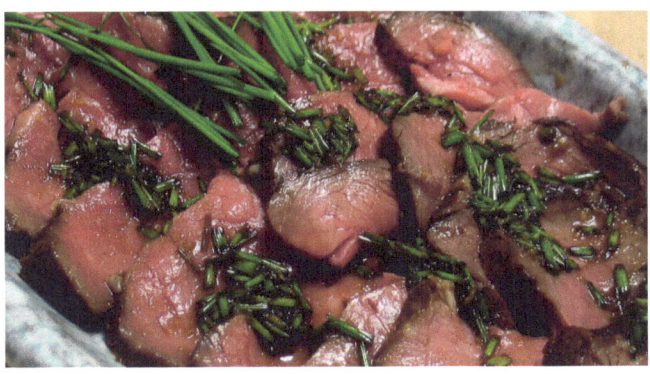

3. Beef Tataki

Tataki is a method of food preparation used by the Japanese where the fish or meat (in this case, beef) is cooked very rare on the inside and seared on the outside to give you that contrasting flavors and textures of fresh and cooked, tender and crispy. You need to slice the meat or fish thinly. Serve this dish with soy sauce flavored with citrus. This special version of Ttataki includes a salad of carrots, radishes, and onions. You can serve this dish as a topping to soba noodles made of buckwheat to turn it into a full meal. This meal takes about 40 minutes to prepare. Image from Flicker by John Ivan

Ingredients:

• A pound of sirloin steak, boneless and trimmed, cut into 1-inch thick
• A cup of red radishes, chopped into sticks (you can also use daikon radish, a kind of radish that is long and white and can be bought from Asian stores and natural or organic food shops)
• A cup of carrots, chopped into sticks
• Half a cup of onions, sliced thinly
• A quarter cup soy sauce, low sodium
• 2 tsp. and 2 tbsp. of freshly squeezed lemon juice
• 2 tbsp. of scallions, chopped finely
• 2 tsp. of fresh ginger, grated finely
•   2 tsp. of canola oil
•   ¼ tsp. of black pepper, freshly ground

Instructions:

1. Soak the onions, carrots, and radishes in a bowl with cold water for about 5 minutes. Drain the vegetables and set aside.

2. In a smaller bowl, mix together the ginger, scallions, lemon juice, and soy sauce. Dress your drained vegetables with a couple of tbsptablespoons of this sauce. Set aside the rest of the sauce for later use.

3. Coat your steak with salt and pepper on both sides to bring out the flavors. Turn on the stove to medium-high heat, place a large nonstick pan over the burner, and add the canola oil. When the oil is hot enough, add the steak and cook for about 3 to 4 minutes on each side if you want your steak to be medium-rare. Once the steak is cooked, place it on a chopping board and let it cook for about 5 minutes. Cut the steak into thin slices and drizzle with the rest of the unused sauce. Serve with your springy salad of carrots, radishes, and onions.

4. Makes 4 servings.

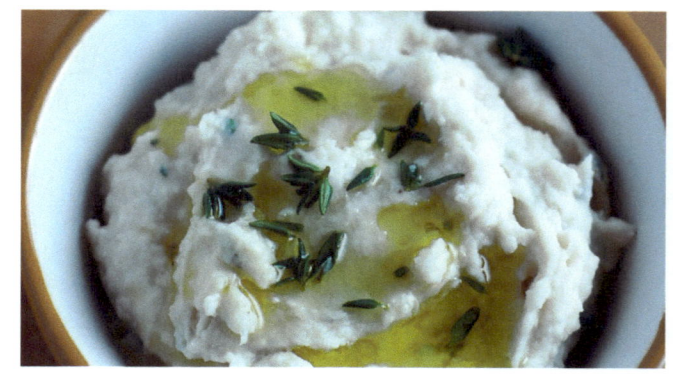

4. Lemon and Thyme Ricotta Dip

Ingredients:

• 1 15 ounce container of fresh, part skim ricotta cheese
• 2 tablespoons of fresh thyme chopped
• 2 tablespoons of shallot, minced or chopped finely
• 1 teaspoon of fresh chives, chopped
• 2 teaspoons of lemon zest
• ¼ cup of freshly squeezed lemon juice
• ½ teaspoon of sea salt
• 1 teaspoon of black or white pepper
• 2 teaspoons of extra virgin olive oil

Instructions:

Using a blender, food processor or regular mixer, whip together the ricotta, thyme, chives, shallots, lemon zest and juice, salt and pepper until light and smooth.

Place in a bowl and drizzle with 2 teaspoons of olive oil. Serve with fresh vegetables, wheat thins, naan or tortilla chips.

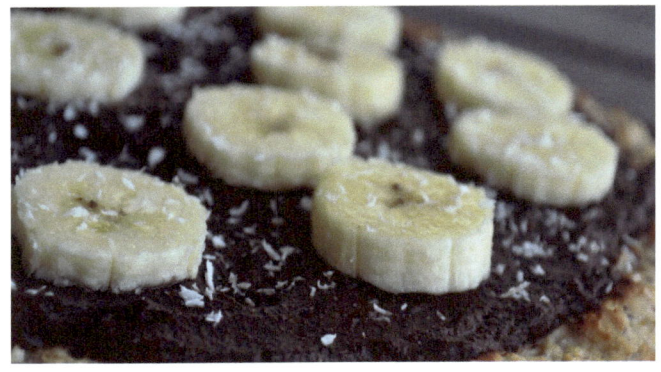

5. Bananas crusted with cocoa and coconut

Scrumptious desserts like this recipe makes the transition from your unhealthy eating habits to a cleaner and greener lifestyle a lot easier. This is perfect for the whole family and can also be served as a snack or breakfast. Total preparation time is only 10 minutes. Image from Flicker by Louise

Ingredients:
• 2 bananas, small and sliced diagonally
• 4 tsp. of cocoa powder
• 4 tsp. of toasted coconut, unsweetened

Instructions:
1. Put the cocoa powder on one plate and the toasted coconut on another. Cover each banana slice with cocoa powder and coconut by rolling them first in the cocoa powder, then dipping them in the coconut.

2. This makes 4 servings.

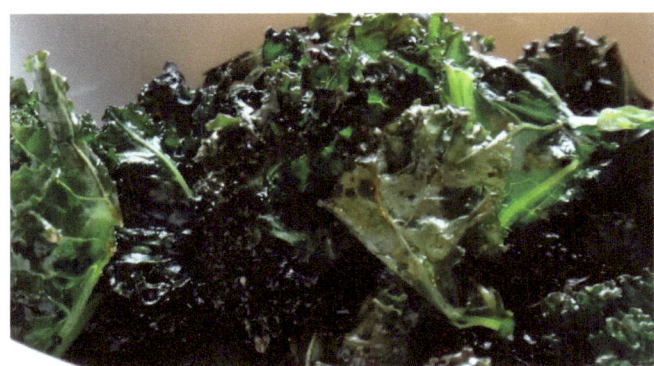

6. Easy Homemade Kale Chips

Ingredients:
• 1 large bunch of fresh kale
• 1 Tablespoon of olive oil
• 1 tablespoon of sherry vinegar
• 1/8 teaspoons of kosher or sea salt

Instructions:
Preheat your oven to 150 degrees Centigrade.

Trim and prep your kale by taking the ribs out of each leaf. Dry the kale and drizzle with olive oil. Toss the leaves by hand to ensure that each is coated with oil. Sprinkle with vinegar and toss well.

Line a baking sheet with a silicone baking sheet or parchment paper and evenly spread the leaves.

Bake for about 35 minutes or until the chips are crispy.

Season with salt and serve as is or with some homemade tartar sauce.

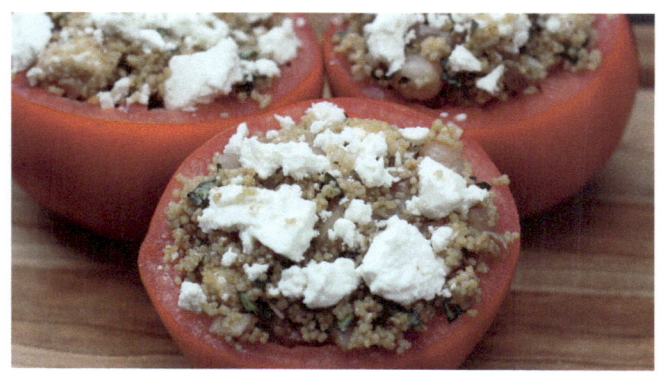

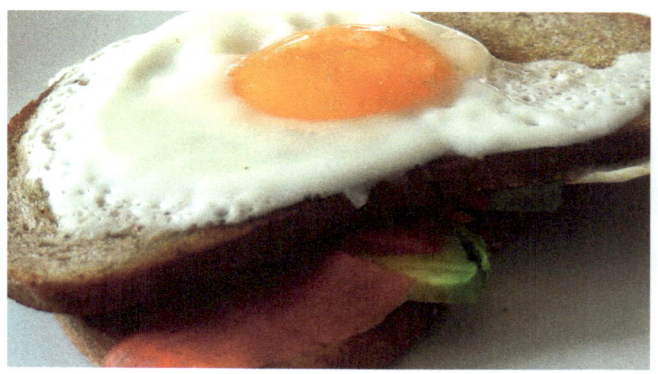

7. Goat Cheese Stuffed Tomatoes

Ingredients:
• 24 pieces of cherry tomatoes
• 3 ounces of fresh goat cheese
• 1 tablespoon of low fat milk
• 2 tablespoons of chopped green or black olives
• 2 teaspoons of chopped oregano (fresh)
• 1/8 teaspoons of pepper

Instructions:
Slice the tops of each cherry tomato and scoop out the seeds (if any). Set aside and start preparing the filling.

Mix the goat cheese, olives, milk, pepper and oregano together to form a paste.

Fill each tomato's cavity and drizzle with olive oil, more oregano and pepper. You can chill these before serving.

8. Salmon and Egg Sandwich

If you need a quick and easy healthy breakfast that will boost your energy in the morning, this power sandwich is what you need. You can get your complex carbohydrates from the English muffin made from whole wheat and your protein and healthy fats from the egg whites and smoked salmon. If you want a heavier breakfast, you can pair this sandwich with a glass of freshly squeezed fruit juice or smoothie and a piece of fresh fruit. It takes about 15 minutes to prepare this sandwich. Image from Flicker by Charles Smith

Ingredients:
• 1 oz. of salmon, smoked
• 1 English muffin, made from whole-wheat flour, sliced into two and toasted
• Egg whites from a couple of large eggs, beaten
• A slice of tomato
• 1 tbsp. of red onion, chopped finely
• ½ tsp. of capers, rinsed and roughly chopped
• ½ tsp. of extra virgin olive oil
• Salt to taste

Instructions:

1. Turn on the stove to medium heat and heat the extra virgin olive oil in a nonstick pan. Cook the onion until tender and translucent, which will take about a minute. It is important to continuously stir the onion to keep them from burning. Cook the capers, salt, and egg whites together with the onions for about half a minute or until the egg whites are set. Be sure to stir continuously. Turn off the stove.

2. Put one slice of the whole-wheat English muffin on a small plate and layer the egg white mixture, smoked salmon, and fresh tomato. Cover with the other half of the muffin.

3. Makes one sandwich.

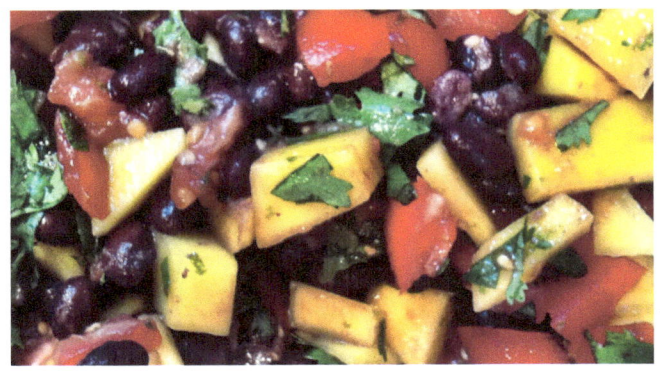

9. Healthy Black Bean Salsa

Ingredients:

• 3 cans or about 3 and ½ cups of black beans. You can buy dried ones and cook them until tender
• 1 cup of Mexican corn or 1 can of corn
• 4 large fresh Roma tomatoes, diced
• 1 large green chili pepper (Jalapeno)
• ½ cup of green onions, chopped
• 1 bunch of cilantro leaves
• Salt and pepper to taste

Instructions:

Mix together all the ingredients, except for the cilantro leaves. If you want the cilantro taste to come together with the rest of the mixture, you may chop half of the bunch and toss it in. Season with salt and pepper.

Place the mixture in a bowl, top with the remaining cilantro leaves and serve with tortilla, corn chips or crackers.

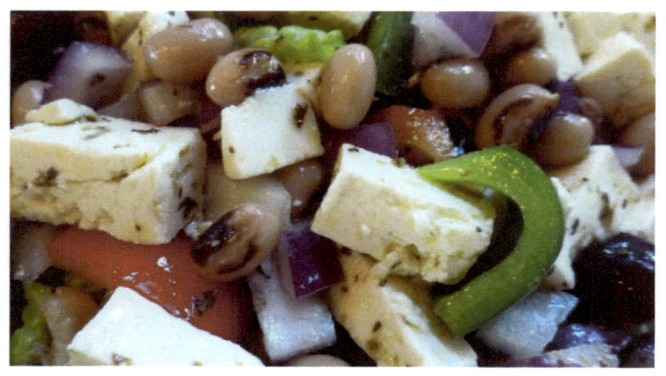

10. Black-Eyed Peas and Cucumber Salad

This is a great side dish with any meat dish. You can serve this salad on a bed of greens like romaine lettuce or arugula. If you do not have black-eyed peas or you prefer other legumes, you can use chickpeas or white beans instead. However, the black-eyed peas add an interesting color to the salad, which makes it look more appetizing. This recipe takes about 20 minutes to prepare. Image from Flicker by Gerald

Ingredients:
• 14 oz. black-eyed peas
• 4 cups of cucumber, peeled and diced
• 2/3 cup of bell pepper, preferably red for that added color
• ½ cup of feta cheese, crumbled
• ¼ cup of red onion, slivered
• 2 tbsp. of black olives, chopped
• 2 tsp. of fresh oregano, chopped, or 1 tsp if dried
• 2 tbsp. of lemon juice, freshly squeezed
• 3 tbsp. of extra virgin olive oil
• Black pepper, freshly ground (to taste)

Instructions:

1 In a large bowl, mix together the black pepper, oregano, and freshly squeezed lemon juice using a whisk to ensure that all the ingredients and well incorporated.

2. Toss in the rest of the ingredients including the black-eyed peas, cucumber, feta cheese, red bell pepper, olives, and onions. Make sure that all the ingredients are well coated with the dressing.

3. You can serve this dish at room temperature or chilled.

4. Makes 6 servings. Each serving is equivalent to about a cup.

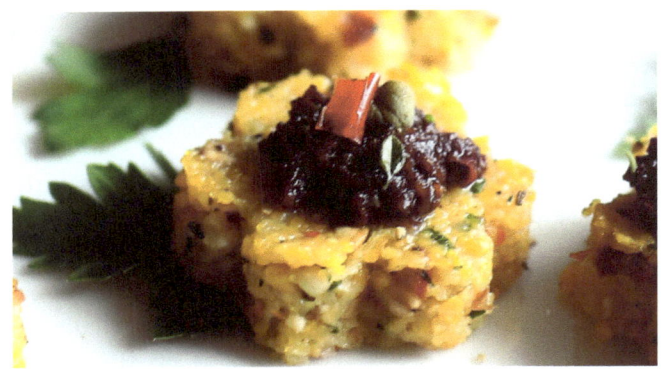

11. Crispy Polenta Wedges with Tomato Tapenade

Ingredients:

• 1 tube of pre-made polenta (you can make your own by cooking polenta on a stove, according to package direction and spread onto a lined baking sheet and chill to solidify.)
• Cooking spray or canola oil
• 2/3 cup of sun dried tomatoes (canned or jarred)
• 4 teaspoons of olive oil
• 1 tablespoon of chopped flat-leaf parsley
• 2 teaspoons of capers, rinsed to remove the excess salt
• 1 garlic clove minced
• 1/8 teaspoons of pepper

Instructions:

Preheat your oven to 350 degrees and line a baking sheet with parchment paper and spray some non-stick cooking spray over the paper. You can also oil the sheet with canola oil.

Slice the polenta into wedges or triangles and place them, evenly spaced, onto the baking pan. Bake the polenta wedges for about 15 minutes or until the edges are crispy and let them cool.

In a food processor, blend the tomatoes, parsley, garlic, olive oil, capers and pepper into a thick but not so smooth paste.

Top each polenta wedge with the tomato tapenade, sprinkle with parsley and serve.

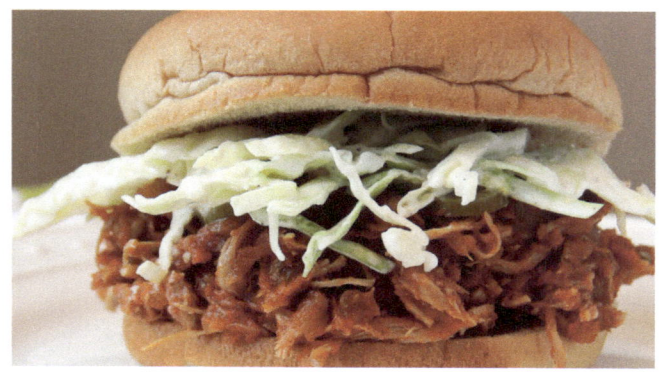

12. Barbecue Pulled Chicken

This is a fancy dinner that you can serve when you have guests at home. It is a version of the pulled pork barbecue. The chicken is cooked slowly to make sure that the meat is tender in a large amount of tomato sauce. This can be a hearty main dish when topped with sour cream, red onions, and jalapenos. It can also be served with spaghetti made from whole-grain or mashed potatoes. Some also use this as filling for their sandwich and as an ingredient to a healthy salad, which includes low fat mayonnaise, honey, seeds of celery, and shredded Nnapa cabbage. This recipe is so simple yet tasty and versatile, which makes up for the long preparation time of 5 and ½ hours. Image from Flicker by Remy67

Ingredients:
• 2 and ½ lb. of chicken thighs, deboned, skinned, and trimmed of fat
• 8 ounce tomato sauce
• 4 oz. green chiles, chopped
• 1small onion, chopped finely
• 1 clove of garlic, minced
• 3 tbsp. of cider vinegar
• 2 tbsp. of raw honey
• 1 tbsp. of Worcestershire sauce
• 1 tbsp. of paprika, smoked or sweet
• 1 tbsp. of tomato paste
• 2 tsp. of mustard, dry
• 1 tsp. of chipotle chile, ground
• ½ tsp. of salt

Instructions:

1. You need to use a 6-quart slow cooker or crock pot for this recipe. Cook the first batch of ingredients in the slow cooker including the chiles, tomato sauce, tomato paste, honey, vinegar, Worcestershire sauce, dry mustard, paprika, ground chipotle, and salt until the mixture is smooth. Once smooth, stir in onion, garlic, and chicken.

2. Slow cook the chicken with the lid on for about 5 hours. When the chicken is cooked, you will notice that it can be easily pulled apart, thus the name of this recipe.

3. When the chicken is tender enough, place it on a chopping board and shred the chicken meat using a fork. Put the shredded chicken back into the sauce, stir to incorporate all the ingredients together, and serve while still hot.

4. This recipe makes 8 servings.

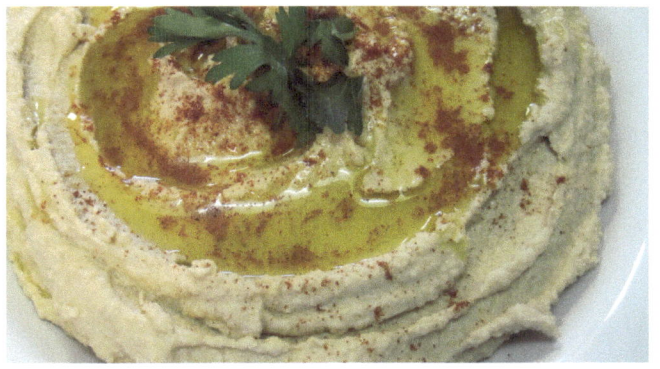

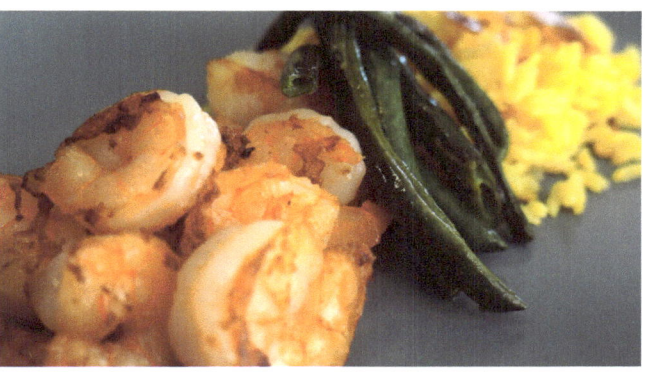

13. Quick and Easy Hummus

Ingredients:

• 1 can or about 15 ounces of cooked garbanzo beans or chick peas
• 2 ounces of fresh Jalapeno peppers, sliced into rounds
• ½ teaspoon of cumin (powder)
• 2 Tablespoons of lemon juice
• 3 large cloves of garlic, chopped

Instructions:

Using a food processor, combine all ingredients together to form a paste. If the mixture is too thick, add a little bit of the chickpea water. Keep adding until you have reached the desired consistency.

Place the hummus in a bowl and serve with sliced flat bread, pita chips or paratha.

14. Saffron Rice and a Gilding of Shrimp

This is a delectable dish that combines different flavors, including the world's most expensive spice, the golden saffron, and other herbs. The summer vegetables add lightness to this dish and the shrimp gives you an ocean flavor that will make you feel like you are vacationing by the Mediterranean Sea. Do not overuse the herbs and spices because the right amount goes a long way. Image from Flicker by Joy

Ingredients:

• 1 lb. or about 21 to 25 pieces of shrimp, peel and vein removed
• A quarter to half a cup of saffron threads
• A cup of brown rice (choose long grain)
• 3 medium-sized yellow summer squash, cut into 4 slices lengthwise and further cut into a quarter inch thick slices
• 1/3 cup of fresh mint leaves, tightly packed in the cup and chopped finely
• 2 and ½ cups of plain water
• 2 tbsp. of freshly squeezed lemon juice
• 2 tbsp. of extra virgin olive oil
• 1 tsp. of salt, to be used separately
• Black pepper, freshly ground, to taste

Instructions:

1. Pour the water in a medium-sized saucepan and add the saffron threads and half a tsp. easpoon of salt. Bring to a boil over medium-high heat. Stir in the brown rice and boil with the cover on. Once the rice and water is boiling, lower the heat and let it simmer. The rice is already cooked when the grains are tender and the water is completely absorbed. This will take about 3 quarters of an hour. You can use a fork to fluff the rice.

2. When the rice is almost cooked, place a nonstick skillet on the stove and heat the olive oil in it. Cook the squash slices for about 5 to 7 minutes or until tender, not brown. Be sure to stir the squash slices to prevent them from burning. Add the shrimp, continue stirring, and cook for about a couple of minutes. Toss in the mint leaves and cook for about half a minute. Stir in the freshly squeezed lemon juice and remove the pan from the burner. Sprinkle with the ground black pepper and remaining salt to taste.

3. Serve this by topping the cooked brown rice with the shrimp and vegetables.

4. Yields 4 servings. One serving is equivalent to a cup of brown rice and 1 and ½ cups of shrimp and vegetables.

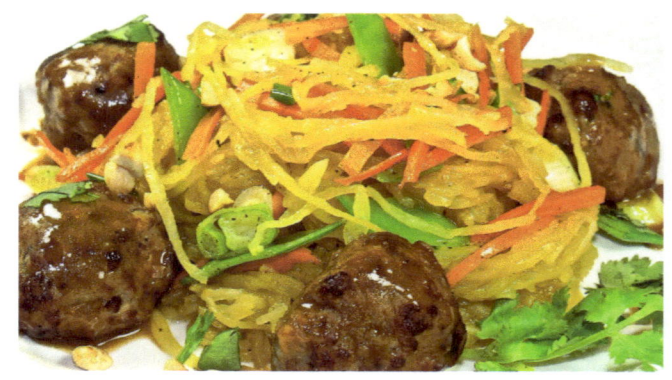

15. Thai-Style Chicken Balls

Ingredients:
- 2 lbs. of minced chicken
- 1 cup bread crumbs
- 4 green onions, chopped
- 1 tablespoons of coriander powder
- 1 cup of fresh cilantro, chopped
- ¼ cup of Thai sweet chili sauce
- 2 tablespoons of freshly squeezed lemon juice
- Canola oil for frying

Instructions:

In a bowl, mix together chicken, bread crumbs, chopped green onions, coriander powder, cilantro, chili sauce and lemon juice together. Form balls out of the mixture and set aside. Chill the prepared chicken balls to make sure that it is firm enough for frying.

Meanwhile, heat oil in a deep pot or fryer. Once the chicken balls are firm enough, fry each ball in hot oil.

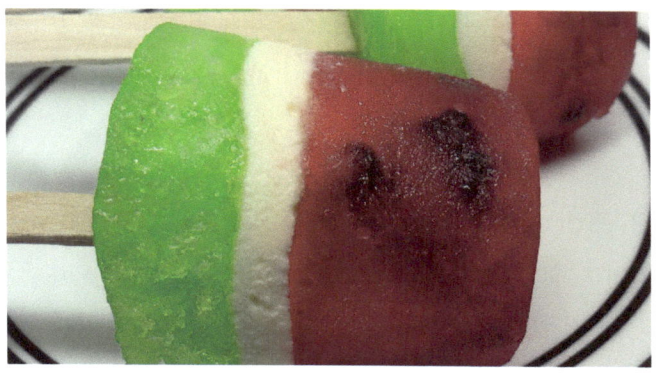

16. Blueberry and Watermelon Ice Pops

This is a healthier version of the frozen fruit pops that you can buy in the grocery. Kids will surely love this, especially the whole blueberries frozen inside the fruit pops, which resemble watermelon seeds. Image from Flicker by Vannessa

Ingredients:
- A cup of fresh blueberries
- 3 and ¾ cups of seedless watermelon, chopped
- 2 tbsp. of lime juice
- 1 to 2 tbsp. of sugar

Instructions:
1. Toss the chopped watermelon, sugar, and lime juice in the food processor and pulse until it reaches a pureed texture.

2. Divide your blueberries evenly among your 10 frozen pop molds, add the watermelon puree, and seal the mold by inserting the sticks. Pop them in the freezer for about 6 hours or until the fruit pop is firm. To easily remove the mold from the frozen fruit pop, briefly dip the molds in hot water.

3. Makes 10 fruit pops.

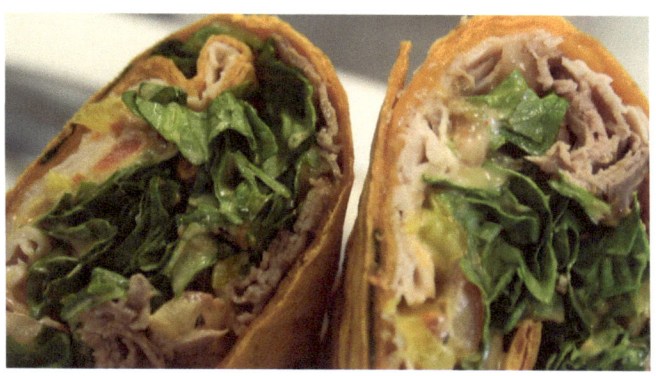

17. Steak and Blue Cheese Wrapped Bell Peppers

Ingredients:
- 16 thinly sliced steak, grilled
- 1 cup of blue cheese or goat's cheese
- 4 large red and yellow bell peppers cut into strips.

Instructions:
Spread a generous amount of cheese onto each steak.

Place about 3 or 4 pepper strips on top of the cheese and roll each piece of steak to form a log. Secure each with a toothpick.

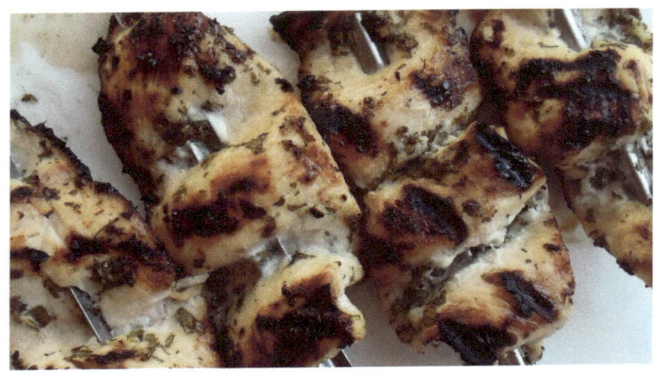

18. Grilled Chicken Tenders with Cilantro and Sesame Seeds Pesto

This is a quick and flavorful dinner that can be made even healthier by serving it with grilled asparagus and quinoa. You can add garlic for that extra flavor if you like. It only takes 35 minutes to cook this dish. Image from Flicker by Cale65

Ingredients:

- 1 lb. of chicken tenders
- 2 cups or about 1 to 2 bunches of fresh cilantro leaves, loosely packed
- 2 tbsp. of sesame seeds, toasted
- 2 scallions, thinly sliced
- A quarter cup of soy sauce, low sodium
- A quarter cup of lime juice
- 1 tbsp. of canola oil
- 1 tsp. of powdered chili

Instructions:

In a large bowl, combine the soy sauce, canola oil, and lime juice using a whisk. Set aside a couple of tbsp. of this mixture in a small bowl for later use. Toss the chicken tenders into the rest of the marinade and make sure that the chicken pieces are coated evenly. You can also use a re-sealable plastic bag instead of bowl to easily coat the chicken with the marinade. Put this inside the fridge for about an hour or so to let chicken tenders soak in the flavors.

2. Turn on the grill at medium-high temperature.

3. Process the cilantro, sesame seeds, scallions, and the 2 tbsp. of marinade that you have set aside in the food processor until mixture is smooth.

4. Get the marinated chicken from the fridge and discard the marinade. Put the chicken on the oiled grill rack and cook for about a couple of minutes on each side or until the chicken is cooked through the middle. Serve the grilled chicken with the pesto made of cilantro and sesame seeds.

5. Makes 4 servings.

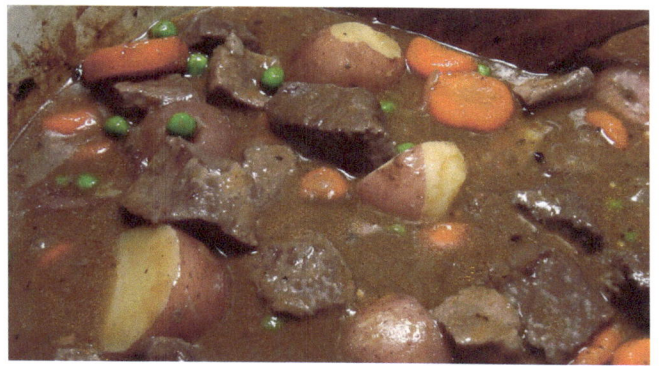

19. Fragrant Stew with Shredded Beef

This is a basic stew with simple ingredients but complex flavors. It uses a part of the beef called the flank steak that has a strong meaty flavor. The flank steak may have a tough texture but it can be tenderized so that the meat can easily be shredded by cooking it in a slow cooker. This is a perfect dish for fall or winter. Image from Flicker by Xavier

Ingredients:

• 3 lbs. of beef flank steak, fat removed and steaks cut into 3 slices each

• 1 and ½ cups of chicken broth, low sodium

• A quarter cup of sherry vinegar

• 1 piece of large bell pepper, preferably red, seeded and chopped

• 1 piece of large onion, chopped

• 2 stalks of celery, roughly chopped

• Half a cup of fresh cilantro leaves, packed and chopped

• Half a cup of pickled jalapenos, chopped

• 10 corn tortillas

• 3 garlic cloves, minced

• 1 tbsp. of cumin, ground

• 1 tsp. of salt

• Half a tsp. of black pepper, freshly ground

Instructions:

1. Pour the chicken broth and vinegar into a 6-quart slow cooker. Add the spices such as the cumin, garlic, bell pepper, onion, celery, pepper, and salt. Stir in the beef, making sure that it is completely submerged by surrounding the beef pieces with the vegetables.

2. Cover the crock pot and cook on low for about 8 hours or until the beef is tender enough when you press a fork in it.

3. When the beef is cooked, transfer to the chopping board and allow to cool for about 10 minutes. Using 2 forks, shred the beef apart and put them back to the crock pot. Add the cilantro. Put the stew in a serving bowl and serve with still warm tortillas and garnish with pickled jalapeno.

4. Makes 10 servings.

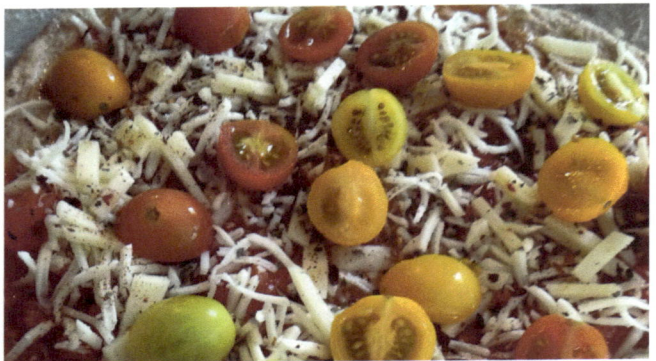

20. Quick Tomato-Mozzarella Pizza

Ingredients:

• 1 frozen whole wheat pizza dough (you can also use large tortillas or flat breads)

• 2 tablespoons of yellow cornmeal or course corn flour

• 5 large plum tomatoes, sliced thinly

• 1 large clove of garlic, minced

• 1 cup of shredded fresh mozzarella cheese

• ¼ teaspoons of black pepper

• ¼ cup of basil, sliced into thin strips

*you can also use bacon or pancetta slices

Instructions:

Preheat your oven to 350 degrees. If you have a pizza stone, you may place the stone in the oven to heat up.

Prepare the dough by sprinkling some cornmeal all over the edges. Sprinkle the rest of the cornmeal onto a baking sheet or your pizza stone.

Spread the minced garlic all over the dough and sprinkle half of the cheese on top. Arrange the tomatoes on top and sprinkle the basil leaves.

Add the rest of the cheese and bake for about 10 minutes or until the cheese has melted. Slice and serve.

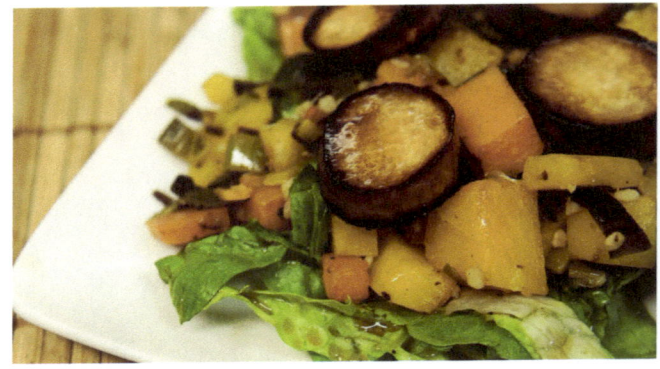

21. Seared Scallops with Sautéed Mushrooms and Leeks

The combination of mushroom and leeks, brandy and sour cream gives this dish a robust flavor. You can also use vermouth instead of brandy if you want a milder flavor. You can also serve the mushroom and leek mixture with poultry or meat. This is best served over barley. Total preparation time is half an hour. Image from Flicker by Ivan

Ingredients:

• 1 lb. of large sea scallops (Note: Choose 'dry' scallops because these scallops have not been subjected to chemical baths, unlike 'wet' scallops. Dry scallops are also firmer and more flavorful than 'wet' scallops' They also brown nicely when cooked.)

• 10 oz. of mushroom, chopped

• 2 cups of leeks, sliced thinly (only use the white and light green parts)

• A quarter cup of brandy or the milder vermouth

• A quarter cup of chicken broth, low sodium

• 3 tbsp. of sour cream, low fat

• 1 tbsp. of fresh parsley, roughly chopped

• Half a tsp. of salt, to be used separately

• Black pepper, freshly ground, to taste

• 4 tsp. of extra virgin olive oil, to be used separately

Instructions:

1. Put a large nonstick pan on the stove and turn on the heat to medium-high. Add half of the olive oil on the pan. Cook the mushroom for about 3 minutes or until they release their natural moisture. Add the leeks and reduce heat to prevent burning. Cook about 8 minutes or until the leeks are almost brown. Continue stirring the vegetables. Pour in the brandy and chicken broth and cook until the liquid thickens, which takes about half a minute. Turn off the stove and add parsley, sour cream a quarter tsp of salt, and black pepper. Put on the lid and set aside.

2. Season the scallops with the remaining half of the salt and black pepper. Heat the remaining half of the oil and cook the seasoned scallop in a nonstick skillet about 2 to 3 minutes or until they turn to golden brown.

3. Pour a generous amount of the mushroom and leek mixture on a plate and top with the cooked scallops.

4. This recipe yields 4 servings.

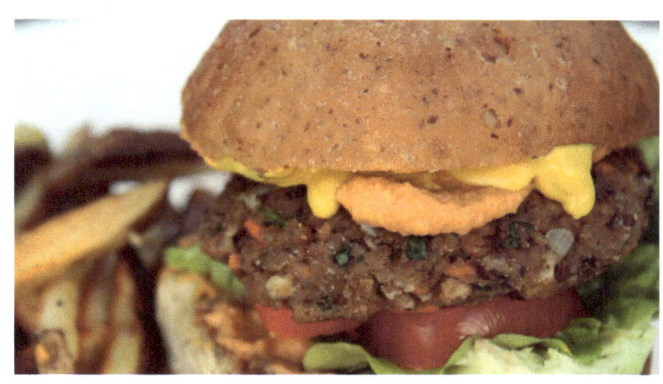

22. Vegetarian Burgers

Ingredients:
- 1 medium sized zucchini, grated
- 1 potato, grated
- 1 medium carrot, grated
- ¼ cup of onions, minced
- ½ teaspoon of chopped oregano
- 2 egg whites or egg replacer equivalent to 2 eggs

Instructions:
Mix all the ingredients together. Make sure that everything has been incorporated well.

Form into patties in your desired size and thickness and place in the chiller to firm up.

Heat a pan with a little bit of cooking oil and fry each patty when firm.

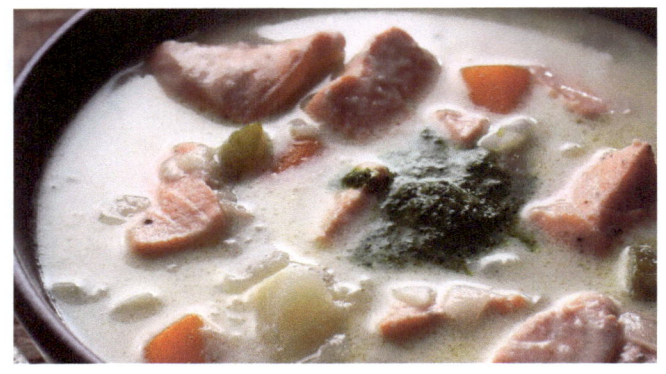

23. Salmon Chowder

Adding dill or tarragon to this chowder recipe gives it a unique flavor. The mashed potatoes give this soup a rich and smooth texture that reminds you of butter or heavy cream. You can also use leftover mashed potatoes but the overall texture will not be as smooth and velvety. Serving this to your whole family will make you feel like it is Christmas morning instead of an ordinary day. You can also add mushrooms and mashed lentils if you like. Total cooking time is about half an hour. Image from Flicker by Joseph

Ingredients:

• 12 oz of salmon fillets, skinned and preferably caught in the wild, like in the Pacific Ocean near Alaska and Washington state
• 2 and ½ cups of cauliflower florets, chopped coarsely
• 1 and 1/3 cups of mashed potatoes
• A quarter cup of fresh dill, chopped, or 2 tsp tarragon, dried
• 1/3 cup of carrots, chopped
• 1/3 cup of celery, chopped
• 3 tbsp. of fresh chives or scallions, chopped, or 1 ad ½ tbsptbsp. of dried chives
• 4 cups of chicken broth, low sodium
• 1 and ½ cups of plain water
• 1 tbsp. of Dijon mustard
• 1 tbsp. of canola oil
• A quarter tsp. of salt
• Black pepper, freshly ground, to taste

Instructions:

1. Use a large saucepan to heat the canola oil. The stove should be set at medium heat. Cook the celery and carrots for about 3 to 4 minutes or until they start to turn golden brown. Stir frequently to prevent burning. Pour in the water and chicken broth and add the cauliflower, chives or scallions, and the salmon fillets. Put on the lid and let it simmer to cook the salmon well. This will take about 5 to 8 minutes. Put the salmon on a chopping board and shred into small chunks using a fork.

2. Add the dill or tarragon, Dijon mustard, and mashed potatoes into the soup. Maintain gentle simmer and return the salmon chunks into the pan. To add flavor, season with salt and pepper.

3. Yields about 6 servings. One serving is equivalent to 1 and ½ cups.

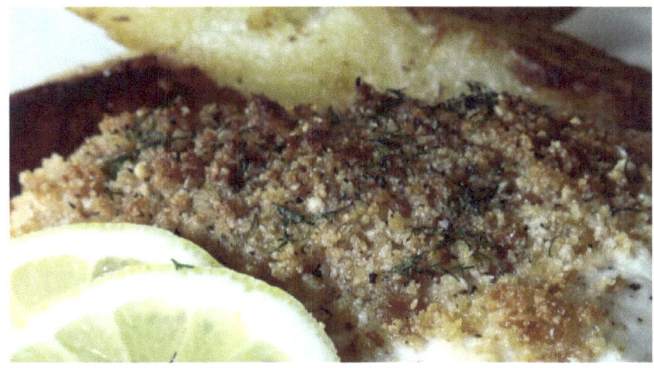

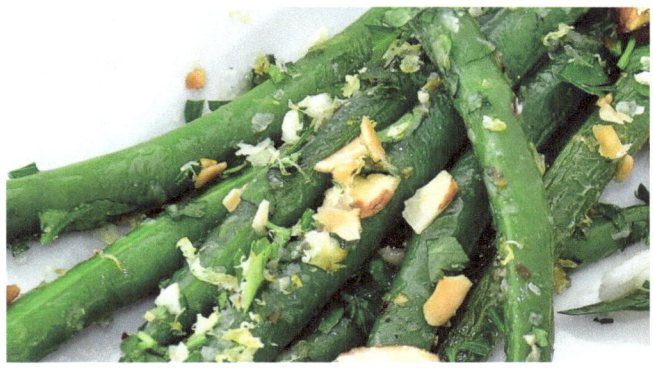

24. Quick Baked Halibut

Ingredients:

- 1 teaspoon of olive oil
- 1 cup medium zucchini, diced
- ½ cup of onion, chopped
- 1 large clove of garlic, grated
- 2 cups of Roma tomatoes, diced
- 2 tablespoons of basil, chopped
- ¼ teaspoon of salt
- ¼ teaspoon of ground black pepper
- 2 halibut steaks
- 1/3 cup of feta cheese, crumbled

Instructions:

Preheat your oven to 450 degrees. Line a baking tray with parchment or baking paper.

In a medium sauce pan, heat olive oil and sauté the garlic, onions and zucchini. Once the zucchini has softened, turn off the heat and stir in the tomatoes, basil and season with salt and pepper.

Place the halibut steaks on the baking sheet and top with the sautéed vegetables. Drizzle with a little bit of olive oil and bake for about 15 to 20 minutes.

25. Green Beans with Dill and Lemon Vinaigrette

Tasty dill and lemon vinaigrette areis the perfect pair for cooked green beans. The vinaigrette is very versatile and can also be used as a dressing to fresh tomato slices and steamed asparagus. It only takes 25 minutes to prepare. Image from Flicker by Kobi

Ingredients:

- 1 lb. of green beans, trimmed
- 1 tbsp. of freshly squeezed lemon juice
- 4 tsp. of fresh dill, chopped
- 1 tbsp. of shallot, minced
- 1 tsp. of mustard, whole-grain
- 1 tbsp. of extra virgin olive oil
- A quarter tsp. of salt
- A quarter tsp. of black pepper, freshly ground

Instructions:

1. Boil water about an inch high in a sauce-pan. Put a steamer basket on top of the pan and place the green beans ion the basket. Put the lid on and steam for about 5 to 7 minutes or until the beans are tender enough but still crispy. Turn off the stove and remove the pan from the burner to stop the cooking process.

2. Get a large mixing bowl and combine the lemon juice, oil, dill, shallot, mustard, salt, and pepper using a whisk. Once these ingredients are well combined, toss in the steamed green beans to coat. Let it sit for about 10 minutes or so to allow the green beans to fully absorb the flavors.

3.   Yields 4 servings. One serving is equivalent to about 1 cup.

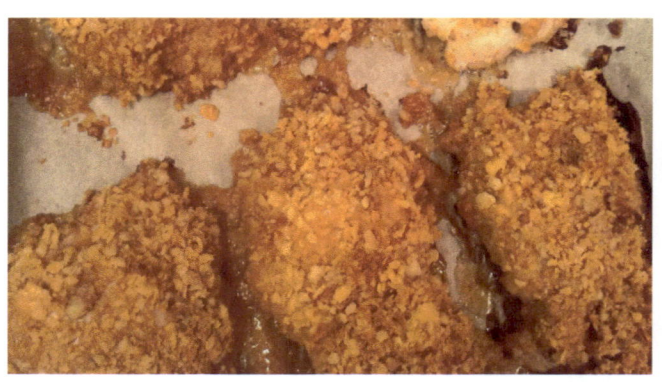

26. Cornflake Crusted Chicken with Pineapple Salsa

Ingredients:
Salsa
•1 cup of chopped fresh pineapple
•2 tablespoons of fresh cilantro leaves, chopped
•1 tablespoon of finely chopped red onion
•Chicken
•1/3 cup of lightly crushed plain corn flakes
•1 cup panko break crumbs or herbed Italian bread crumbs
•½ teaspoon of salt
•A pinch of pepper
•4 large chicken cutlets or chicken breast fillet (skinless)
•1 ½ teaspoons of canola oil for frying, add more if you are using a non-stick pan

Instructions:
 Make the salsa first by combing all the ingredients together. Place in an air tight container and refrigerate.

Combine cornflakes. Salt, pepper and bread crumbs in a small bowl. You can add other herbs such as cilantro, parsley and even paprika. Coat each cutlet with the cornflake mixture and set aside.

Chill the chicken cutlets and heat your pan.

Fry the chicken pieces until golden brown. You may bake the chicken fillets in a 450 degree oven for about 15-20 minutes. Serve oin a platter with some pineapple salsa on the side.

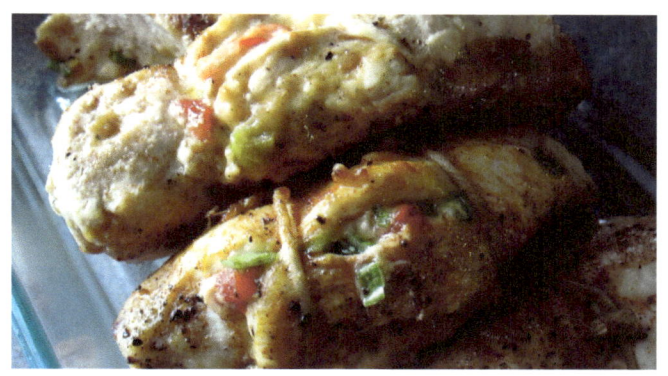

27. Cheese Pimiento-Stuffed Chicken Breasts

To add a unique flavor to plain chicken breasts, you can stuff them with ingredients such as cheese, pimientos, and scallions, like this recipe. This does not require too much effort on your part but the outcome is delicious. The filling might ooze out while the chicken is cooking in the oven but this is okay—just scoop out the spilled filling from the pan for a cleaner presentation. This is best served with sautéed vegetables like summer squash with barley or zucchini. Image from Flicker by Jimmy

Ingredients:

•4 small (about 1 ¼ to 1 ½ lb.) chicken breasts, boneless and skinless, removed tenders and trimmed

•Half a cup of Gouda cheese, shredded (it would be better if the cheese is smoked)

•1 tbsp. of pimientos, sliced

•2 tbsp. of scallions, chopped

•1 tsp. of paprika, to be used separately

•1 tbsp. of extra virgin olive oil

•Half a tsp. of salt, to be used separately

•Half a tsp. of ground pepper, to be used separately

Instructions:

1. Preheat the oven at a temperature of 400 degrees F.

2. In a small mixing bowl, mix together your pimientos, scallion, cheese, and half of your paprika.

3. Cut a long slit on the side of each chicken breast from one end to the other. The chicken breast should open like a book. Season the chicken with half of the salt and pepper. Divide the cheese-pimiento-scallion mixture among the 4 breasts. Close the filled chicken breasts by firmly pressing the edges using your fingers. Season the breasts some more with the rest of the salt, pepper, and paprika.

4. Get a large ovenproof pan and put it on the stove over medium-high temperature. Heat the olive oil and place the chicken. The chicken will cook for about a couple of minutes on one side. When the bottom side is already golden brown, flip the chicken breasts over and put the skillet with the chicken into the oven. Bake the chicken for about 15 minutes or until the thermometer reads 165 degrees F when inserted into the thickest portion of the chicken or when the center of the chicken is cooked through.

5. Makes 4 servings.

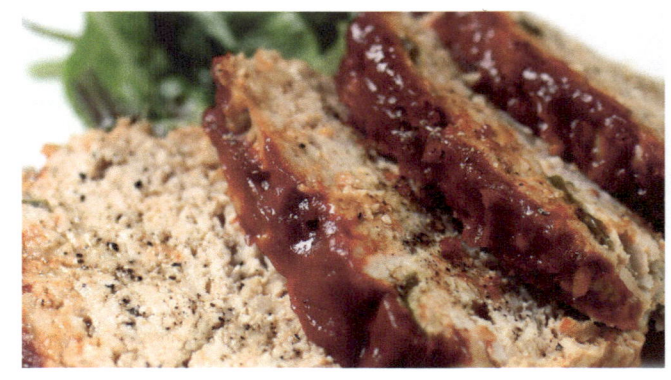

28. Lean and Healthy Meatloaf

Ingredients:

• 1 lb turkey breast, minced

• 1 lb of lean beef, minced

• ¼ cup of sun dried tomatoes or about 2 tablespoons of tomato paste

• 1 cup of red onion, diced

• 1 cup bell pepper, finely chopped

• ½ cup of carrot, diced finely

• 1 cup of zucchini, grated

• ¼ cup of chopped parsley

• 2 whole eggs

• ½ teaspoon of fresh thyme

• 4 large cloves of garlic, crushed

• ½ cup of panko bread crumbs

• ¼ cup ground flaxseed

• ¼ teaspoon of pepper, salt

• ¼ cup of organic chicken broth

Instructions:

Preheat your oven to 350 degrees and grease a large loaf pan with baking spray or canola oil. You can line it with parchment paper as well.

Mix all the ingredients together until well combined.

Place the mixture in the prepared pan and bake for about 1 ½ to 2 hours. Watch over the meatloaf because it can dry out easily, since you will be using turkey and lean meat. If using a meat thermometer, the center of the meatloaf should be within the 150 to about 170 degrees.

Let the cooked meatloaf rest and cool off a bit before unmolding and slicing.

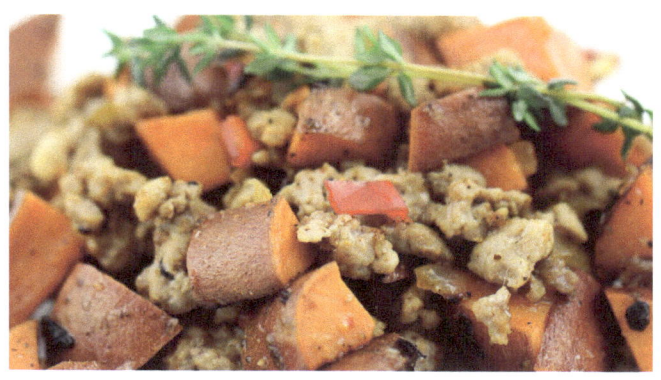

29. Turkey and Sweet Potato Hash

Hash is a great way to use leftover meat and transform it into a new dish. This recipe combines the different flavors of sweet potatoes, onions, apples, and turkey. Image from Flicker by Dennis

Ingredients:

•3 cups of turkey (or chicken), skinless, cooked, and diced

•2 medium-sized sweet potatoes, chopped into ½-inch thick slices

•1 medium-sized apple, cored and chopped into ½-inch thick slices

•1 medium-sized onion, chopped

•Half a cup of sour cream, low fat

•1 tbsp. of canola oil

•1 tbsp. of fresh thyme, chopped, or 1 tsp. when dried

•1 tsp. of freshly squeezed lemon juice

•Half a tsp. of salt

•Black pepper, freshly ground, to taste

Instructions:

1. Boil sweet potatoes in a medium-sized saucepan. Once boiling, lower the heat and continue cooking for about 3 minutes. Toss in the chopped apple and cook for about a couple of minutes or so, making sure that they are tender enough but not mushy. Discard water when cooked.

2. Get 1 cup of the apple-sweet potato mixture and mash it in a large bowl. Add the lemon juice and sour cream. Stir in the rest of the apple and sweet potato mixture. Set aside.

3. Cook onion in a nonstick skillet with hot olive oil for about a couple of minutes or so. Stir in the turkey, salt, pepper, and thyme. Occasionally stir. Cook for about a couple of minutes.

4. Stir in the mashed sweet potato and apple into the turkey and stir. To cook the hash, press the mixture using a wide spatula to brown the bottom. This will take about 3 minutes. Using your spatula, cut the hash into sections. Turn it over to cook the other side for another 3 minutes. Best served while still hot.

5. Yields 6 servings, about 1 and ¼ cup each serving.

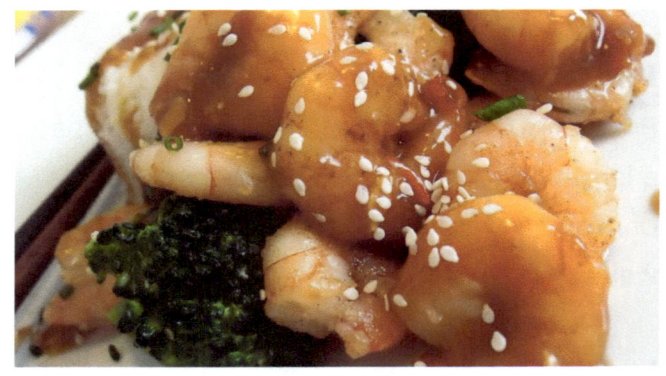

30. Szechwan Shrimps

Ingredients:

- 12 ounces of medium shrimps – peeled, deveined and butterflied
- 4 cloves of garlic, chopped
- ¼ cup chopped green onions
- ¼ teaspoon ginger powder
- 1 tablespoon of ground nut oil/ peanut oil
- ½ teaspoon of red pepper flakes
- 2 tablespoons of ketchup
- 4 tablespoons of water
- 1 tablespoon of tamari or light soy sauce
- 1 teaspoon of honey or agave
- 2 teaspoons of cornstarch

Instructions:

Prepare the sauce by mixing all the wet ingredients together. Add in the red pepper flakes, cornstarch and ground ginger and stir well.

In a large wok, heat oil and sauté the garlic and green onions until fragrant. Add the shrimps and cook until they are almost cooked and immediately stir in the sauce mixture.

Wait until the shrimps are fully cooked and the sauce has thickened before turning off the heat. Serve with cooked brown rice.

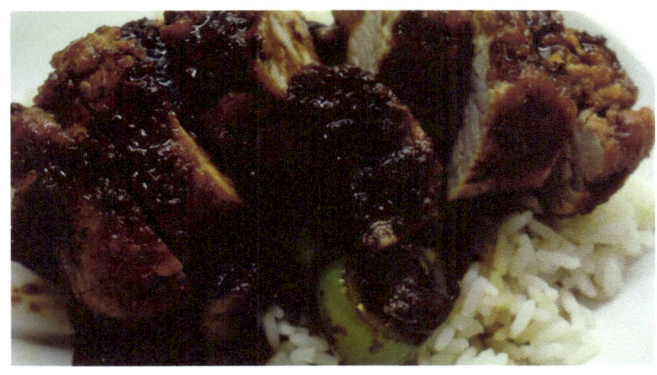

31. Pork Tenderloin with Mustard and Maple Sauce

Pork tenderloin is a healthy meat option because it is lean. The maple and mustard sauce gives this dish and sweet and savory flavor. You can add sage, rosemary, or thyme to give it a delicious twist that your taste buds will surely love. Image from Flicker by Barry

Ingredients:

• 1 lb. of pork tenderloin, trimmed of fat

• 2 tbsp. of maple syrup

• 3 tbsp. of Dijon mustard, to be used separately

• A quarter cup of cider vinegar

• 1 and ½ tsp. of fresh sage, chopped

• 2 tsp. of canola oil

• Half a tsp. of kosher salt

• Half a tsp. of black pepper, freshly ground

Instructions:

1. Preheat the oven at a temperature of 425 degrees F.

2. In a small bowl, mix together salt, pepper, and 1 tbsp. of Dijon mustard. Rub the pork tenderloin with this mixture. Cook the tenderloin in hot oil using an ovenproof skillet. The pork will cook for about 3 to 5 minutes, making sure that all sides are brown. Put the skillet into the oven and bake the pork for about 15 minutes or until the thermometer reads 145 degrees F when inserted into the middle of the pork. Put the roasted pork on a chopping board and let it cool for about 5 minutes.

3. Put the skillet on the stove at medium-high heat and boil the cider vinegar for about half a minute. Scrape up the browned bits at the bottom of the skillet using a wooden spoon to prevent burning and for added flavor. Stir in the maple syrup and the rest of the Dijon mustard. When boiling, lower the heat and keep it simmering for about 5 more minutes or until the sauce is thick enough.

4. Cut the pork into thin slices and add the sage and pork juices to the sauce. Pour the sauce over the pork and serve.

5. Makes 4 servings.

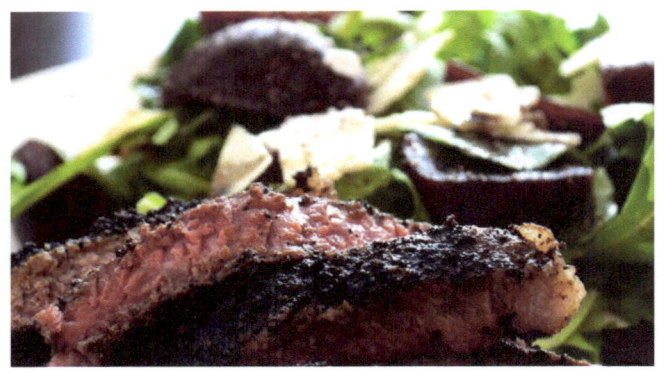

32. Cumin and Coriander Crusted Steak

Ingredients:

•1 tablespoon of brown sugar, packed

•1.2 teaspoon of salt

•½ teaspoon of pepper

•½ teaspoon of cumin powder

•½ teaspoon of coriander powder

•¼ teaspoon of red pepper powder

•1 lb. boneless sirloin steak

Instructions:

Preheat your oven to 450 degrees. Coat a thick oven safe pan or cast iron skillet with oil and place it inside the oven to heat up.

Combine all the ingredients together and rub all over the prepared steak.

Place the steak in the pan and bake for about 7 minutes for medium cook. Slice thinly, against the grain.

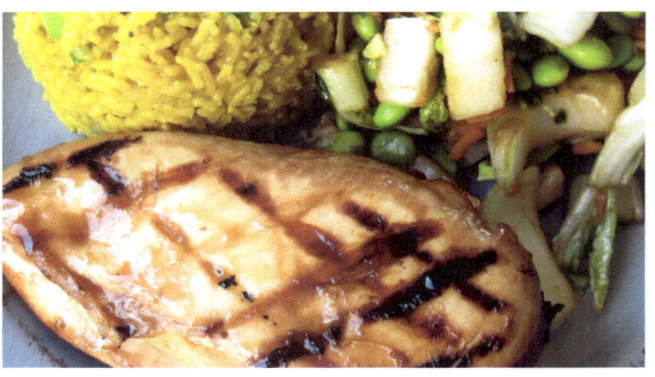

33. Hawaiian Chicken

Ingredients:

•2 pieces of large chicken breast fillet

•¼ teaspoon each of the following spices:

o Ginger

o Paprika

•¾ teaspoon of onion powder

•1 ½ teaspoon of garlic powder

•1 tablespoon of apple cider vinegar

•¼ cup of tomato sauce

•1 tablespoon of soy sauce or tamari

•1 5 ounce can of crushed pineapple

•½ tablespoon of brown sugar

•Cooked brown rice

Instructions:

Preheat your oven to about 400 degrees and line a baking sheet with parchment paper.

Place the chicken fillets in the pan and set aside.

Mix together the onion, garlic, paprika and ginger powders and add in the vinegar. Baste the top of the chicken with the mixture and bake for about 10 minutes.

After 10 minutes, turn the chicken and baste the top with the remaining vinegar mixture and place it back in the oven.

In a small bowl, mix the remaining ingredients together except the brown rice. Coat the chicken fillets with the ketchup and pineapple mixture and bake for another 15 minutes or until the chicken fillets have formed crusts. Serve on top of a plate of cooked brown rice.

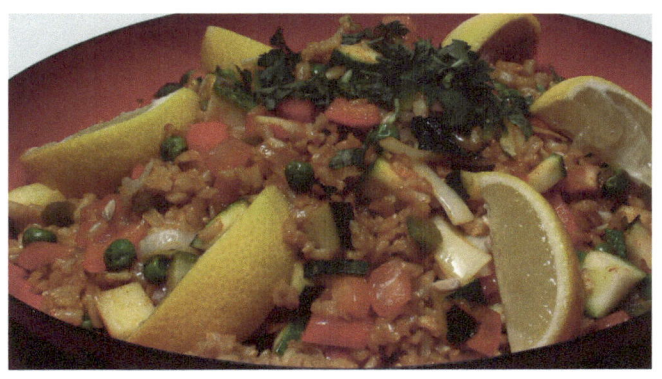

34. Stir-Fry Chicken with Lemon

This colorful stir-fry is a great lunch for the whole family. It is made even more flavorful because of the lemony zest. Image from Flicker by Larry

Ingredients:
• 1 lb. of chicken breasts, boneless and skinless, trimmed and chopped into 1-inch thick slices
• Half a cup of chicken broth, low sodium
• 1 piece of lemon
• A cup of carrots, diagonally sliced at about a quarter inch thick
• 2 cups or about 6 oz. of snow peas (remove the stems and strings)
• A bunch of fresh scallions, chopped into 1-inch thick slices (divide the green and white parts)
• 10 oz. of mushrooms, chopped in halves or quarters
• 3 tbsp. of soy sauce, low sodium
• 1 tbsp. of canola oil
• 2 tsp. of cornstarch
• 1 tbsp. of garlic, chopped

Instructions:

1. Get a tsp. of lemon zest by grating the skin of fresh lemon and set aside. Squeeze the pulp with your hands to get 3 tbsp. of lemon juice. Mix together lemon juice, soy sauce, cornstarch, and chicken broth in a mixing bowl.

2. Place a skillet on the stove at medium-high temperature ad heat the canola oil. Cook the chicken breasts for about 4 to 5 minutes. When cooked, put the chicken on a plate. Cook the carrots and mushrooms in the same pan for about 5 minutes or until tender. Stir in the white parts of the scallion, snow peas, lemon zest, and garlic. Continue stirring for about half a minute until fragrant. Pour the broth mixture into the pan and cook for 2 to 3 minutes, stirring, until the mixture thickens. Toss in the green parts of the scallion, the chicken, and any juices from the chicken and cook for about a minute or two.

3. Makes 4 servings. One serving is equivalent to 1 and ½ cups.

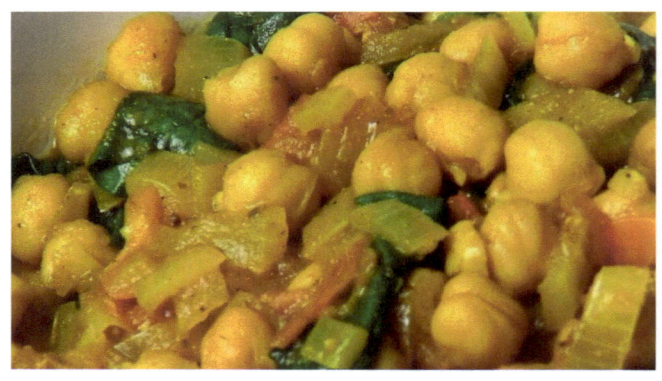

35. Healthy Chickpea Curry

Ingredients:
•2 cans or 2 cups of cooked garbanzo beans or chickpeas
•2 T of vegetable oil
•2 red onions, chopped
•2 large cloves of garlic, crushed
•2 teaspoons of fresh ginger, grated
•6 whole cloves
•2 sticks of cinnamon
•1 teaspoon of ground cumin
•1 teaspoon of ground coriander
•Salt to taste
•1 teaspoon of cayenne pepper
•1 teaspoon of turmeric powder
•1 cup of chopped cilantro
•½ cup Vegetable stock

Instructions:
Heat oil in the pan and sautesauté all your aromatics (garlic, onions and ginger) until fragrant. Add in your spices and fry the mixture until you can smell all the spices.

Stir in the garbanzo beans and sautesauté for about 5 minutes.

Add the stock and simmer for 10 to 15 minutes. Adjust seasoning to taste. Top with fresh cilantro leaves.

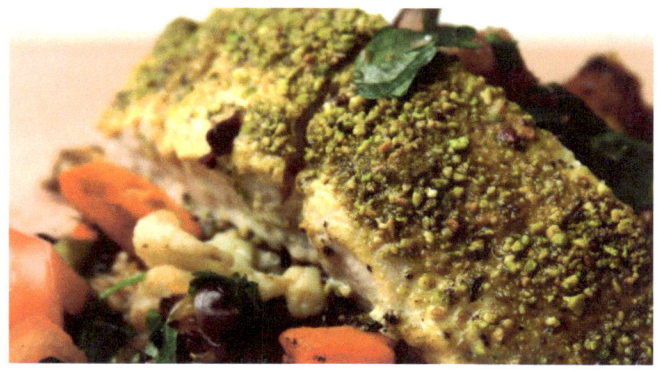

36. Tuna Steaks Crusted with Pistachio

The combination of the flavors and texture of pistachio and dill-mustard sauce makes this tuna dish exceptional. Image from Flicker by Justin

Ingredients:

•4 tuna steaks (about 4 oz. each)

•Half a cup of white wine

•A quarter cup of pistachios, shelled

•A quarter cup of breadcrumbs, coarse and dry

•2 tsp. of fresh dill, to be used separately

•1 tsp. of mustard, whole-grain

•3 tbsp. of sour cream, low fat

•1 bay leaf

•1 tbsp. of shallot, sliced thinly

•2 tsp. of freshly squeezed lemon juice

•Half a tsp. of salt, to be used separately

•A tsp. of extra virgin olive oil

Instructions:

1. Bring the wine, shallot, and bay leaf to a boil in a saucepan. Cook until wine is almost completely reduced, which takes about 5 minutes. Turn off the stove and transfer the contents to a bowl. Discard the bay leaf. Stir in the lemon juice, a tsp. of dill, a quarter tsp. of salt, mustard, and sour cream.

2. Process the pistachios, remaining dill and salt, and breadcrumbs in the food processor until ground finely. Put this powdered mixture in a bowl and coat the tuna steaks with this mixture.

3. Cook the dredged tuna in hot oil until brown, which will take about 4 to 5 minutes on each side. Serve the pistachio-crusted tuna with your lemon-dill-mustard sauce.

4. Makes 4 servings.

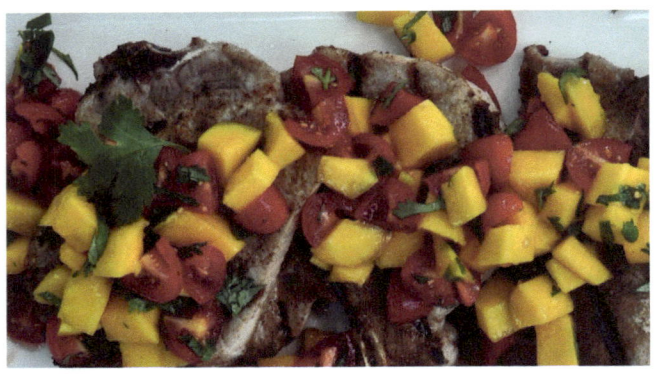

37. All-Spice Pork Chops with Mango Salsa

Ingredients:

- ¾ teaspoon of chili powder
- ¼ teaspoon of sea salt
- 1/8 teaspoon of all- spice powder
- 4 medium sized pork chops (de-boned)
- 1 and a half cups of diced mangoes (ripe)
- 2 tablespoons of fresh mint, chopped
- 1 tablespoons of lemon juice (fresh)
- 2 teaspoons of sugar
- ¼ teaspoons of red pepper flakes

Instructions:

Prepare the marinade for the pork. Mix together the all- spice powder, salt and chili powder. Evenly coat the pork with the spice blend and chill for about 20 minutes.

Heat a skillet and add oil. Once the chops are ready, pan fry each chop, about 4 to 5 minutes per side or until cooked evenly.

While waiting for the pork to cook, prepare your salsa by combining the rest of the ingredients. Chill the mango salsa.

Place 2 pieces of chops per plate and top with mango salsa to serve.

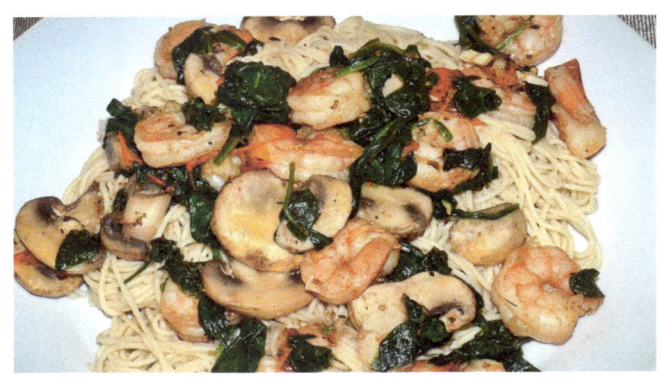

38. Tomato and Spinach Angel Hair Pasta

Ingredients:

- 1 cup of vegetable stock
- 12 pieces of sundried tomatoes
- 2 tablespoons of toasted pine nuts
- ¼ teaspoon of crushed red pepper flakes
- 1 large clove of garlic, crushed
- 1 bunch of fresh spinach leaves, torn into bite size pieces.
- ¼ cup parmesan cheese, grated
- 8 ounces of angel hair pasta, cooked according to package direction
- Salt and pepper to taste

Instructions:

In a large sauce pan, sauté garlic and red pepper flakes until fragrant. Add in the spinach and sun dried tomatoes and cook until the tomatoes have soften. Pour the broth and simmer for about 4 minutes.

Add the cooked pasta, toss in the pine nuts and simmer until the pasta has absorbed the sauce. Mix well and serve. Sprinkle with parmesan cheese.

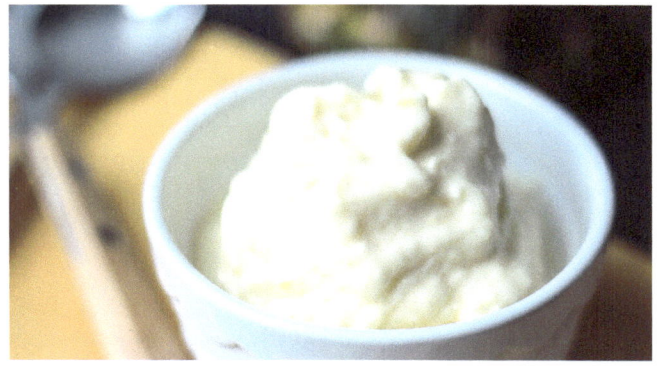

39. Healthy and Light Frozen Peanut Butter Yogurt

Ingredients:

•2 cups of plain or vanilla flavored yogurt – none or low fat yogurt works too!

•½ cup milk (dairy or non-dairy)

•½ cup peanut butter or any nut butter of your choice

•1 ½ teaspoon of pure vanilla extract

•¼ teaspoon of sea salt

•1/3 cup of natural sugar (agave/maple)

Instructions:

In a food processor or blender, mix together all the ingredients until thoroughly combined.

Place in individual cups, ramekins or air tight containers and freeze. Top with crushed cacao nibs, crushed peanut butter cups or cookies before serving.

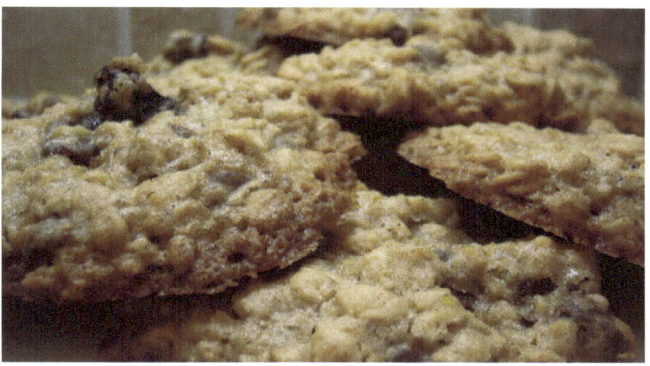

40. Date and Oatmeal Cookies

Ingredients:

•2 large ripe bananas

•5 large Medjool pitted dates

•2 cups of rolled oats – gluten free

•Pinch of cinnamon and sea salt

Instructions:

Preheat your oven to 350 degrees and line a baking pan with parchment or baking paper.

Using a food processor, blend the oats until it reaches a coarse texture. Add in the dates and blend. Add the bananas and the rest of the ingredients to form a dough.

Scoop out the dough and make about 1 inch balls. Place them evenly on the prepared tray and bake for about 17 minutes. Let the cookies cool before serving.

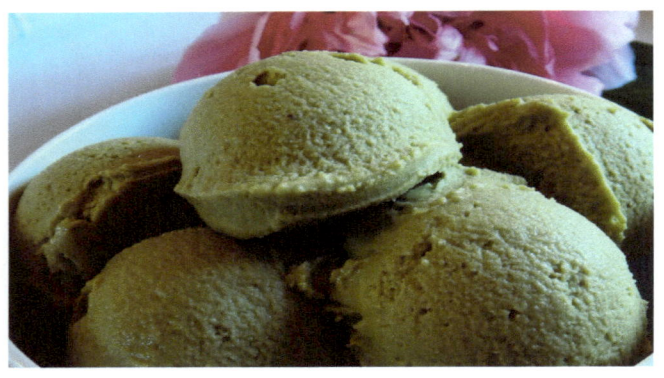

41. Non-Dairy Avocado Ice Cream Tropicale

Ingredients:

•2 large ripe avocados, pitted and sliced

•1 can (15 ounces) pineapple bites, reserve the juice

•½ cup of coconut milk

•3 Tablespoons Fresh Lime Juice

•A pinch of sea salt

•½ cup of raw cocoa powder

•½ coconut oil

•¼ cup of maple syrup

Instructions:

Spread the avocado and pineapple slices onto a baking sheet and freeze for 3 hours.

Process the frozen fruits until the mixture forms a smooth paste and then slowly add the lime juice, pineapple juice, coconut milk, salt and vanilla. Place the mixture in an air tight or covered bowl and freeze until needed.

While waiting for the avocado ice cream to freeze, prepare the chocolate shards or chips.

Melt the coconut oil (if solid) and add the cocoa powder. Mix well before adding the maple syrup. Pour the mixture in a lined pan and freeze to solidify.

Run the avocado mixture in your ice cream maker to churn. It may take about 20 minutes.

Scoop out the ice cream in bowls and garnish with chocolate shards.

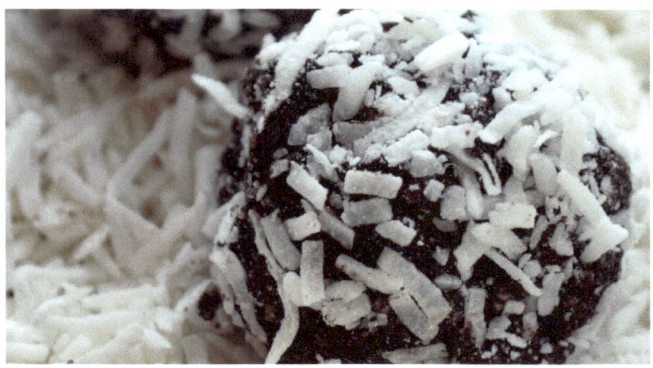

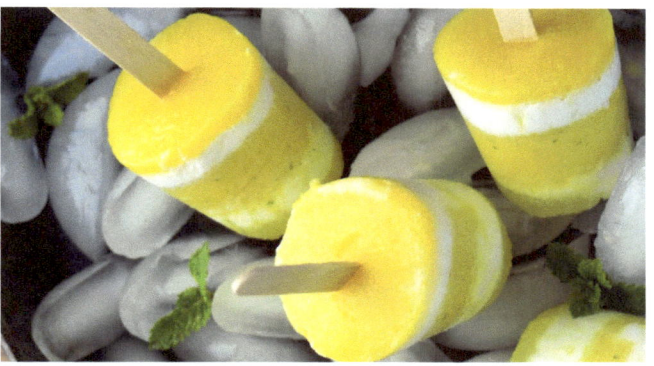

42. No-Bake Healthy Coconut Snow-Balls

Ingredients:

•1 ¾ cups unsweetened coconut shreds, divided plus a little bit of extra

•2 teaspoons coconut oil, melted

•3 tablespoons of maple syrup

•½ teaspoon vanilla

•½ teaspoon cinnamon powder

•1/8 teaspoon of salt

Instructions:

In a food processor, blend together 1 cup of the coconut shreds and the coconut oil until the mixture turns into a paste.

Add the maple syrup, vanilla, cinnamon and salt. Once incorporated, mix in the rest of the coconut shreds. The mixture will be doughy but not firm.

Form the dough into balls and dredge them in the remaining coconut flakes. Chill for about an hour.

43. Mango-Colada Popsicles

Ingredients:

•2 cups frozen mango (organic)

•¾ cup unsweetened coconut milk

•1 cup unsweetened full fat coconut cream/ milk

•1 and half tablespoons of honey or agave or coconut nectar for vegans

Instructions:

Puree the frozen mango and add about ¼ cup of the unsweetened coconut milk.

In a small bowl, add the rest of the coconut milk, 1 cup of the canned coconut cream and your chosen sweetener.

Prepare your Popsicle molds. Pour 2 table-spoons of mango puree into the molds, let it set for a bit and pour the creamy mixture on top. Cover the molds and insert the sticks. Freeze solid.

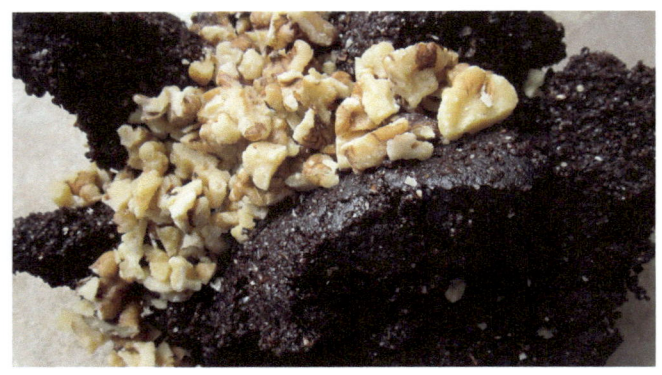

44. Raw Brownies

Ingredients:

•1 cup raw pecans or walnuts

•1 cup Medjool dates, pitted

•5 tablespoons of raw cacao or raw cocoa powder

•2 tablespoons of agave nectar, maple syrup or honey

•¼ teaspoon sea salt

Instructions:

In a food processor, grind the pecans until it becomes coarse, add the dates. As soon as the mixture becomes sticky, it is now ready for the rest of the ingredients.

Blend the rest of the ingredients and pour the mixture ion a lined baking sheet. Spread evenly and refrigerate for at least 3 hours.

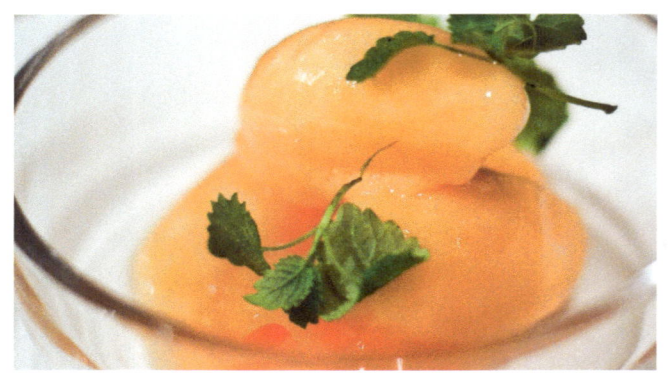

45. Melon and Apple Granita

Ingredients:

•4 cups of ripe melon, cubed

•1 cup unsweetened apple juice (bottled or fresh)

•¼ cup fresh lime juice

•1 cup blueberries (fresh)

•1 cup raspberries (fresh)

•Mint leaves for garnish

Instructions:

Blend all ingredients together (except the mint leaves) and pour the liquid mixture into a shallow pan.

Place the pan in the freezer and let the mixture siet for about 3 to 4 hours. Take the pan out and scrape the slightly frozen mixture. Place it back in the freezer.

Do it again after an hour and let it freeze again. Take the granita out 30 minutes before serving. Scoop the granite into cups and garnish with mint leaves.

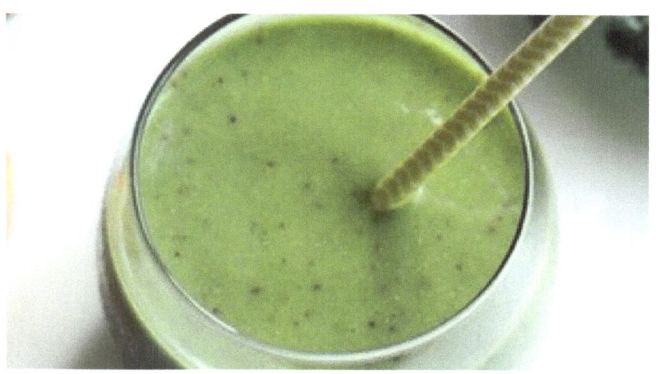

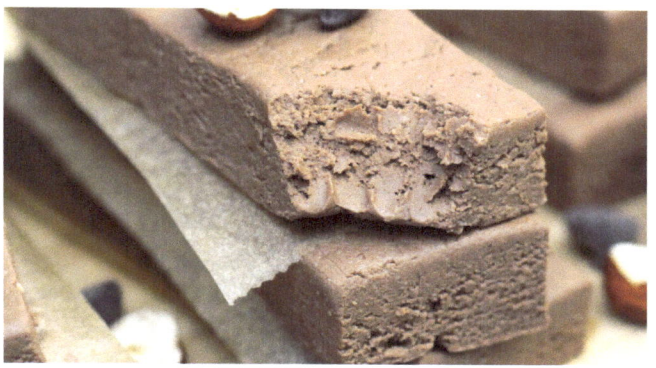

46. Healthy Peachy Green Smoothie

Ingredients:

•2 cups of frozen peaches (if using fresh, freeze them first for about 4 hours)

•2 cups of spinach leaves

•1 cup of water

•1 tablespoon of grated fresh ginger

•1 tablespoon of honey or agave

Instructions:

Pour water, honey, ginger and spinach in a blender and pulse. The mixture should be smooth and really green.

Add the frozen peaches and blend until it forms a smoothie-like consistency.

Serve in chilled tall glasses.

47. Super Healthy Vegan Nutella

Ingredients:

•2 cups of raw hazelnuts

•1 ½ cups of melted dark chocolate

•1/3 cup raw coconut sugar

•1 tablespoon coconut oil

•1 teaspoons of vanilla extract

•¾ teaspoon of salt

Instructions:

Blend the raw hazelnuts into a fine paste and add the rest of the ingredients.

Store the prepared hazelnut spread in a jar and store in the fridge.

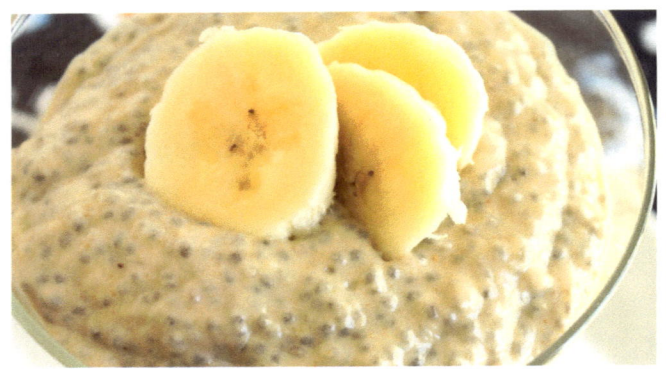

48. Banana Pudding Pots

Ingredients:

•10 pieces of raw almonds- roasted

•2 tablespoons of cornstarch

•a pinch of salt

•3 tablespoons of raw coconut or palm sugar

•1 beaten egg yolk

•¾ cup of milk (dairy or non-dairy)

•½ teaspoon of vanilla extract

•2 ripe bananas, sliced thinly

•6 dessert cups

Instructions:

In a food processor, grind the almonds and set aside.

In a small pot, mix together sugar, cornstarch and salt. Add the egg yolk and slowly pour the milk. Heat the mixture until it thickens.

Remove the pan from the heat and add the vanilla. Let it cool slightly.

Prepare the cups by placing a layer of the sliced bananas, topped with the custard cream mixture. Create another layer of bananas and cream until the entire cup has been filled. Sprinkle the chopped almonds. You can choose to serve them cold or warm.

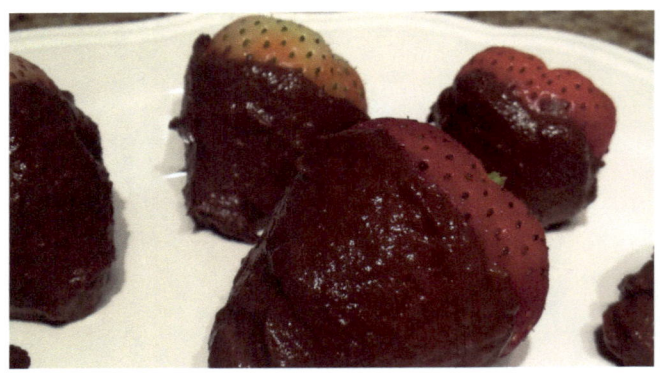

49. Sugar Free Chocolate Covered Strawberries (Paleo)

Ingredients:

•½ kilos of fresh strawberries, cleaned and patted dry

•1/3 cup of pure cacao powder

•1 teaspoon of vanilla bean paste

•A pinch of salt and a teaspoon of honey

•3 tablespoons of coconut oil, melted

Instructions:

Line a baking sheet with parchment paper.

In a small bowl, combine cocoa powder, vanilla bean paste, melted coconut oil, salt and honey.

Dip each strawberry into the chocolate mixture and place on the parchment lined pan.

Chill or let it set in at room temperature.

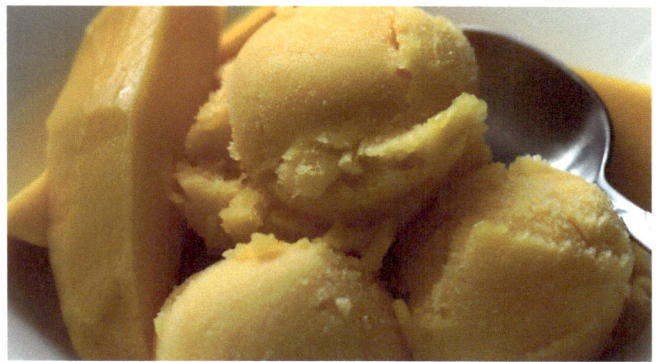

50. Mango, Banana and Pineapple Sorbet

Ingredients:

•1 cup frozen pineapples

•2 cups frozen mango chunks

•4 bananas, room temperature

•4 Tbsp. raw honey, maple syrup, or stevia

•1 Tbsp. fresh lime juice

Instructions:

1. Combine the pineapples, mango chunks, two bananas, honey, maple syrup or stevia, and lime juice in a blender or food processor. Blend until creamy.

2. Spoon the mixture into two small mugs. Slice up two bananas and add them on top. Serve immediately.

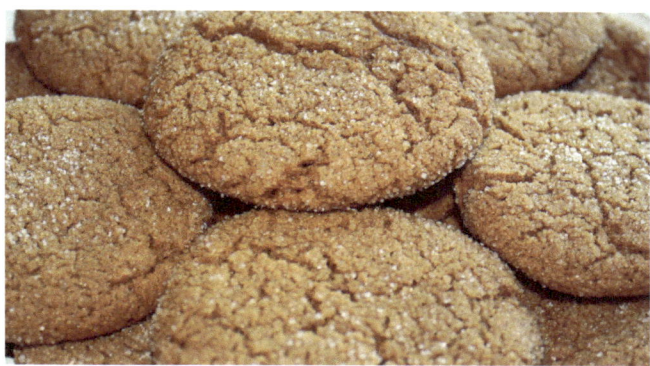

51. Ginger Spice Cookies

Makes: 2 dozen cookies

Ingredients:
•4 cups whole almonds

•4 Tbsp. chia seeds

•2 eggs

•1/2 cup coconut oil

•6 Tbsp. freshly grated ginger

•4 Tbsp. ground cinnamon

•1 tsp nutmeg

•1/3 cup raw honey or maple syrup

•Salt

Instructions:
1. Preheat the oven to 350 degrees F. Line a baking sheet with parchment paper.

2. Combine the almonds and chia seeds in a food processor or blender and process until combined. Pour into a mixing bowl.

3.   Add the eggs, coconut oil, ginger, cinnamon, nutmeg, raw honey or maple syrup, and a pinch of salt into the mixing bowl. Mix well.

4. Using your hands, shape the dough into 24 small balls and line them up on the prepared baking sheet.

5. Bake for 15 minutes, then set on a wire rack to cool before you serve.

CONCLUSION

Clean eating is not that difficult to follow, with all these amazing recipes, tips and guidelines, the only thing that you are left to do is to put everything that you have learned here into action. And once you have gotten used to this really simple, healthy and clean lifestyle, you will be able to achieve that energized and fit body that you have always wanted.

I hope this book was able to help you to understand the basic principles of clean eating and plan your meals for the first week.

The next step is to apply what you have learned in this book when you start the clean eating program.

This book hopes that you will keep all the principles mentioned here in mind – from choosing to buy unprocessed whole foods, to cutting back on your sugar intake – because at the end of the day, your main goal is not just to lose those extra pounds, but to also influence and encourage others to take on the clean eating lifestyle.

Did You Like Clean Eating?

Before you go, we'd like to say "thank you" for purchasing our book. So a big thanks for downloading this book and reading all the way to the end. Now we'd like ask for a *small* favor. Could you please take a minute or two and leave a review for this book on Amazon

This feedback will help us continue to write the kind of Kindle books that help you get results. And if you loved it, then please let me know

Leave a review for this book on Amazon by searching the title: **Say No to Processed Food!** A clean eating recipe book that will give you a healthier life.

Check Out My Other Books

Below you'll find some of my other popular books that are popular on Amazon. Search the titles in Amazon or you can visit my author page on Amazon to see other works done by me.

www.ravenspress.com/jjlewisbooks

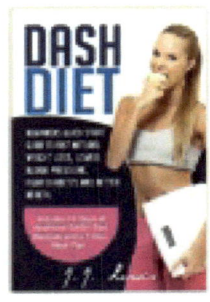 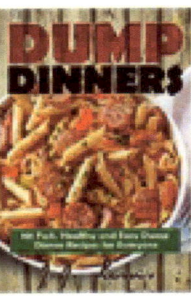 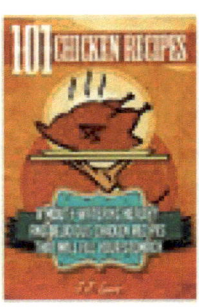 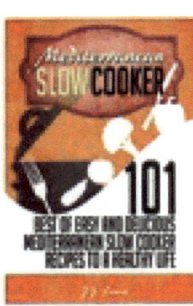 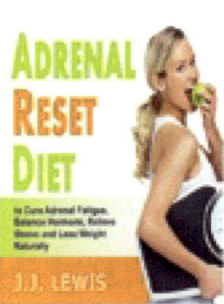

Dash Diet: Beginners Quick Start Guide to Fast Natural Weight Loss, Lower Blood

Dump Dinners: 101 Fast, Healthy and Easy Dump Dinner Recipes for Everyone

Adrenal Reset Diet: 51 Days of Powerful Adrenal Diet Recipes to Cure Adrenal Fatigue, Balance Hormone, Relieve Stress and Lose Weight Naturally

Mediterranean Slow Cooker: 101 Best of Easy and Delicious Mediterranean Slow Cooker Recipes to a Healthy Life

101 Chicken Recipes: A Mouth-Watering Healthy and Delicious Chicken Recipes that will fill your Stomach

Paleo Slow Cooker: 101 Quick and Easy Paleo Recipes for Healthy Life and Weight

101 Pork Chop Recipes: Extraordinary and Delicious Pork Chop Recipes for Everyday Meals

101 Vegetarian Recipes: Top Vegan Diet Recipes to Live a Healthy Lifestyle

Ketogenic Diet: 101 Days of Ketogenic Diet, Low Carb Recipes for Maximum Weight Loss Benefits

Pressure Cooker Recipes: 101 Mouthwatering, Delicious, Easy and Healthy Pressure Cooker Recipes for Breakfast, Lunch, Dinner in 30 Minutes or Less!

Vegan Cookbook: Vegan Diet for Beginners to a Healthy Everyday Life (Vegan Appetizers and Soups Series)

Paleo Diet: 101 Days of Easy Paleo Diet Recipes Made for Beginners to Maximize Weight Loss

Paleo Diet for Kids: A Fun Pack of 101 Flavorful and Energy-Boosting Paleo Recipes Best In Shaping Healthier, Stronger and Happier Paleo-Nourished Kids

Slow Cooker Recipes: The Best of 101 Nutritious and Delicious Healthy Slow-Cooking Recipes for your Crock Pot

The Juice Cleanse: 101 Healthy Juicing Recipes for Weight Loss

Fast Metabolism Diet Recipes: 101 Best of Metabolism Boosting Recipes to Lose Weight Fast
Low Fat Recipes: 101 Incredible Quick & Easy Recipes for a Low Fat Diet
Gluten Free Diet: 101 Delectable and Healthy Gluten-Free Recipes for better lifestyle
Diabetes Diet: 101 Healthy Diabetes Recipes to Reverse Diabetes Forever and Enjoy Healthy Living for Life
Wheat Belly Diet: 101 Days of Grain Free Recipes for an Optimum Belly Diet and Weight Loss

Want more FREE Bestselling Cook Books?

Join my **V.I.P** List now!

I will be giving away Healthy and Delicious Recipes for **FREE!**

Yes, you heard me right! COMPLETELY FREE to everyone just by being a loyal reader!

www.ravenspress.com/jjlewis/

www.ingramcontent.com/pod-product-compliance
Lightning Source LLC
Chambersburg PA
CBHW041513280526

45792CB00004B/1241